Medicine
and Moral
Philosophy

Medicine and Moral Philosophy

A *Philosophy & Public Affairs* Reader

Edited by MARSHALL COHEN, THOMAS NAGEL, and THOMAS SCANLON

Contributors

KENNETH J. ARROW

LAWRENCE C. BECKER

CHRISTOPHER BOORSE

ALLEN BUCHANAN

CHARLES M. CULVER

NORMAN DANIELS

JOEL FEINBERG

PHILIPPA FOOT

BERNARD GERT

MICHAEL B. GREEN

LOREN E. LOMASKY

JAMES L. MUYSKENS

PETER SINGER

STEPHEN P. STICH

DONALD VANDEVEER

DANIEL WIKLER

Princeton University Press
Princeton, New Jersey

Medical ethics.

The essays in this book appeared origina
in the quarterly journal *Philosophy &
Public Affairs,* published by Princeton
University Press.

Christopher Boorse, "On the Distinction
between Disease and Illness," *P&PA* 5,
no. 1 (Fall 1975), copyright © 1975
by Princeton University Press; Lawrence
Becker, "Human Being: The Boundaries
of the Concept," *P&PA* 4, no. 4 (Summe
1975), copyright © 1975 by Princeton
University Press; Michael B. Green and
Daniel Wikler, "Brain Death and Person
Identity," *P&PA* 9, no. 2 (Winter 1980),
copyright © 1980 by Princeton Universit
Press; Norman Daniels, "Health-Care
Needs and Distributive Justice," *P&PA* 1
no. 2 (Spring 1981), copyright © 1981
by Princeton University Press; Loren E.
Lomasky, "Medical Progress and Nation
Health Care," *P&PA* 10, no. 1 (Winter
1981), copyright © 1981 by Princeton
University Press; Kenneth J. Arrow,
"Gifts and Exchanges," *P&PA* 1, no. 4
(Summer 1972), copyright © 1972 by
Princeton University Press; Peter Singer
"Altruism and Commerce," *P&PA* 2, no
(Spring 1973), copyright © 1973 by Prin
ton University Press; Stephen P. Stitch,
"The Recombinant DNA Debate," *P&PA*
no. 3 (Spring 1978), copyright © 1978 b
Princeton University Press; James L.
Muyskens, "An Alternative Policy for
Obtaining Cadaver Organs for Trans-
plantation," *P&PA* 8, no. 1 (Fall 1978)
copyright © 1978 by Princeton Universit
Press; Bernard Gert and Charles M.
Culver, "Paternalistic Behavior," *P&PA*
no. 1 (Fall 1976), copyright © 1976 by
Princeton University Press; Allen
Buchanan, "Medical Paternalism," *P&P*
7, no. 4 (Summer 1978), copyright © 1
by Princeton University Press; Donald
VanDeVeer, "The Contractual Argumen
for Withholding Medical Information,"
P&PA 9, no. 2 (Winter 1980), copyrigh
1980 by Princeton University Press; Joe
Feinberg, "Voluntary Euthanasia and th
Inalienable Right to Life," *P&PA* 7, no.
(Winter 1978), copyright © 1977 by the
Tanner Lecture Trust; Philippa Foot,
"Euthanasia," *P&PA* 6, no. 2 (Winter
1977), copyright © 1977 by Philippa Fo

CONTENTS

PART I.
CONCEPTUAL ISSUES

CHRISTOPHER BOORSE — *On the Distinction between Disease and Illness* — 3

LAWRENCE C. BECKER — *Human Being: The Boundaries of the Concept* — 23

MICHAEL B. GREEN & DANIEL WIKLER — *Brain Death and Personal Identity* — 49

PART II.
HEALTH AND SOCIAL POLICY

NORMAN DANIELS — *Health-Care Needs and Distributive Justice* — 81

LOREN E. LOMASKY — *Medical Progress and National Health Care* — 115

KENNETH J. ARROW — *Gifts and Exchanges* — 139

PETER SINGER — *Altruism and Commerce* — 159

STEPHEN P. STICH — *The Recombinant DNA Debate* — 168

JAMES L. MUYSKENS — *An Alternative Policy for Obtaining Cadaver Organs for Transplantation* — 187

PART III.
MEDICAL PATERNALISM

BERNARD GERT & CHARLES M. CULVER — *Paternalistic Behavior* — 201

ALLEN BUCHANAN — *Medical Paternalism* — 214

DONALD VANDEVEER — *The Contractual Argument for Withholding Medical Information* — 235

PART IV.
EUTHANASIA

JOEL FEINBERG   *Voluntary Euthanasia and the*
Inalienable Right to Life   245

PHILIPPA FOOT   *Euthanasia*   276

INTRODUCTION

Recent years have witnessed a remarkable quickening of interest on
the part of doctors and lawyers, private citizens and government officials in the moral questions raised by the practice of medicine and the
arrangements society makes for the provision of health care. Philosophers and other theorists have taken up these questions in an increasingly important and influential literature. The present anthology,
drawn from articles published over the last decade in *Philosophy &
Public Affairs*, is intended to make available to a wider audience what
we believe are some of the most lucid and penetrating discussions of
these problems.

The first section of the anthology is devoted to the discussion of conceptual issues. In the practice of medicine, and in the legal issues to
which it gives rise, certain concepts that define significant boundaries
have occasioned extensive debate. The most notable are the concepts
of disease (especially mental disease), of death, and of the beginning
of human life. The essays by Christopher Boorse, by Lawrence Becker,
and by Michael Green and Daniel Wikler deal with these issues from a
philosophical standpoint. They are all concerned to distinguish different kinds of boundaries—moral, social, legal, statistical, biological,
and metaphysical—which are too easily confused in the design of
policy. In particular, they emphasize that biological definitions alone
will not support moral principles. They point out, however, that this is
not necessarily a reason to substitute morally based definitions for
biological ones. The relations between the categories—between, for
example, biological definitions and moral principles—have to be examined with care. Boorse's article investigates the normative significance of the socially important concepts of disease, illness, and normality. Rejecting the widely held view that health and disease are
evaluative notions, Boorse argues that health can be defined in purely
descriptive terms, as can disease, which must be distinguished from

the essentially evaluative notion of illness. In the light of these definitions he discusses both the medical status of homosexuality and the
relation of mental illness to legal responsibility. Becker proposes a biological standard for determining when a human being begins to exist
and ceases to exist. He opposes the "brain death" or irreversible coma
criterion for death, but argues that the question of when to withdraw
life support is an independent one. Green and Wikler defend a form of
the brain death criterion on the basis of recent philosophical theories
about what it is for a particular *person* (as opposed to a particular organism) to continue—or cease—to exist. According to the theory they
accept, a person ceases to exist when the causal processes that normally underlie that person's psychological continuity and connectedness
are destroyed. This leads Green and Wikler to the conclusion that, for
normal human beings at least, the irreversible cessation of upper brain
functioning constitutes the death of the person. While their conclusion
does not itself rest on moral premises its adoption would have an effect, which Green and Wikler discuss, on moral and legal arguments
about the withdrawal of medical care from irreversibly comatose patients.

The essays in the second section of the anthology are concerned
with moral principles governing health-care policies and the institutions that give them effect. Norman Daniels's article starts from the
widely shared belief that as a matter of social justice the provision of
basic health care has an especially strong claim on social resources.
Daniels seeks to explain why this is so, and his explanation builds on
the notion of fair equality of opportunity that is central to Rawls's
theory of justice. Like education, he argues, health care—which has
as its aim the maintenance of normal species functioning—must be
available to all who need it if fair equality of opportunity is to be
achieved.

Loren Lomasky does not think that we possess a specific right to
health care or to a national health service. Health care is one among
other interests or needs and is best provided by a medical marketplace
in which people can choose services for themselves in whatever quantity they desire or can afford. If we think that society should provide a
"minimally decent standard" of health care, Lomasky would prefer

that this be done by a system of cash grants or vouchers rather than through the mechanism of a national health service.

Kenneth Arrow also places strong emphasis on the importance of the market mechanism. His article is a consideration of Richard Titmuss's *The Gift Relationship: From Human Blood to Social Policy*. In it Arrow rejects Titmuss's arguments for the moral and even the technical superiority of the voluntary, unpaid system of securing human blood that is established in the United Kingdom. Arrow doubts that the creation of a market in human blood, or a mixed system like that now existing in the United States and in Japan, would in fact decrease the altruism expressed in the donating of human blood. Arrow also doubts many of the arguments that Titmuss gives for believing that the British system of giving may actually increase the efficiency of the economic system.

Peter Singer defends Titmuss against a number of Arrow's arguments. In particular, he emphasizes Titmuss's claim that a voluntary system fosters attitudes of altruism and reinforces the desire to relate to and help others. Arrow prefers to rely on the market to supply the needed blood and regards altruism as a scarce resource. Singer replies that altruism is not, like oil, a scarce resource, the more of which we use the less we have. Rather it increases as it is used and the need for it is perceived more clearly.

Stephen Stich considers the philosophical and moral problems involved in developing an acceptable attitude toward the conduct of recombinant DNA research which, although it promises great benefits to human health and welfare, is also attended by great risks. He rejects both the policy of unqualified freedom of research and the policy of a total ban on such research. For him the crucial question is, How can the risks and benefits be usefully weighted? He investigates problems concerning the estimation of probabilities, the application of cost-benefit analysis, and the choice of moral principles involved in trying to answer the question. He rejects the tempting reliance on a straightforward utilitarian moral principle and suggests a more formal principle that permits freedom of inquiry until the balance of negative over positive consequences reaches a critical point at which we would revert to a utilitarian calculation.

James Muyskens considers the moral problems involved in trying to obtain organs (such as kidneys) for transplantation. He proposes a policy of routine salvaging which, he argues, need not infringe on rights of self-determination or religious freedom. Muyskens rejects the arguments against such a policy put forward by writers like Paul Ramsey and Robert Veatch, and he argues that it is rational to relinquish our right to be buried intact in order to make life-enhancing and life-saving cadaver organs available.

The essays in section three take up the difficult issue of medical paternalism. The relationship between patient and medical practitioner is naturally conceived as an unequal one: marked generally by greater knowledge on the part of the practitioner and frequently by diminished capacity—in extreme cases even unconsciousness—on the part of the patient. Situations thus often arise in which practitioners take themselves to be permitted, or even obligated, to act for the sake of what they believe to be the patient's good despite the fact that this may involve acting without the patient's consent or even contrary to what is known of the patient's wishes. Bernard Gert and Charles Culver argue—against accepted definitions of paternalism—that such behavior can be properly called paternalistic even though it does not involve coercion or interference with the patient's liberty of action. They defend a revised definition of paternalism which gives that notion a widened application in the medical realm. Allen Buchanan's article is concerned with one particular form of behavior that would count as paternalistic under this definition: the withholding of medical information from patients (or, in some cases, from their families) on the ground that they will be better off without it. Buchanan examines several justifications for this practice and finds them inadequate. One of these is the idea that the implicit contract between patient and physician authorizes the physician to minimize harm to the patient by whatever means the physician deems necessary, including the withholding of information. Replying to Buchanan, Donald Van-DeVeer points out that a contractual argument for withholding information can sometimes be compelling. It can be reasonable to authorize a physician to withhold information if the physician decides it is in one's interest, VanDeVeer argues, and when such authorization has been given, it is not paternalistic for the physician to act in accordance with it.

The final section of the anthology investigates the difficult issue of euthanasia. Joel Feinberg argues that the inalienable right to life, interpreted as a discretionary rather than a mandatory right, is not infringed by voluntary euthanasia. He believes that this interpretation of the right to life is very likely the account that best renders the actual intentions of Thomas Jefferson and the other founding fathers when they spoke of a right to life. Philippa Foot distinguishes between voluntary and involuntary, active and passive euthanasia. She argues that nonvoluntary euthanasia (killing a man against his will and without his consent) is never justified. Euthanasia of this type infringes a man's right to life and is therefore contrary to justice. She argues, however, that all the other combinations, nonvoluntary passive euthanasia, voluntary active euthanasia, and voluntary passive euthanasia, are sometimes compatible with both justice and charity. Foot also discusses the difficulties involved in legalizing euthanasia even in those cases where moral principles do not rule it out.

M.C., T.N., T.S.

PART I
Conceptual Issues

CHRISTOPHER BOORSE   On the Distinction
between Disease
and Illness

In this century a strong tendency has developed to debate social issues
in psychiatric terms. Whether the topic is criminal responsibility,
sexual deviance, feminism, or a host of others, claims about mental
health are increasingly likely to be the focus of discussion. This
growing preference for medicine over morals, which might be called
the *psychiatric turn*, has an obvious appeal. In the paradigm health
discipline, physiological medicine, judgments of health and disease
are normally uncontroversial. The idea of reaching comparable cer-
tainty about difficult ethical problems is an inviting prospect. Unfortunately our grasp of the issues that surround the psychiatric turn
continues to be impeded, as does psychiatric theory itself, by a fundamental misunderstanding of the concept of health. With few exceptions, clinicians and philosophers are agreed that health is an essentially evaluative notion. According to this consensus view, a value-free
science of health is impossible. This thesis I believe to be entirely
mistaken. I shall argue in this essay that it rests on a confusion between the theoretical and the practical senses of "health," or in other
words, between disease and illness.

Two presuppositions of my whole discussion should be noted at the
outset. The first is substantive: with Szasz and Flew, I shall assume
that the idea of health ought to be analyzed by reference to physio-

I thank the Delaware Institute for Medical Education and Research and the
National Institute of Mental Health (Grant RO3 MH 24621) for support in
writing this essay.

logical medicine alone.[1] It is a mistake to view physical and mental health as equally well-entrenched species of a single conceptual genus. In most respects, our institutions of mental health are recent offshoots from physiological medicine, and their nature and future are under continual controversy. In advance of a clear analysis of health in physiological medicine, it seems an open question whether current applications of the health vocabulary to mental conditions have any justification at all. Such applications will therefore be put on probation in the first two sections below. The other presupposition of my discussion is terminological. For convenience in distinguishing theoretical from practical uses of "health," I shall adhere to the technical usage of "disease" found in textbooks of medical theory. In such textbooks "disease" is simply synonymous with "unhealthy condition." Readers who wish to preserve the much narrower ordinary usage of "disease" should therefore substitute "theoretically unhealthy condition" throughout.

I. NORMATIVISM ABOUT HEALTH

It is safe to begin any discussion of health by saying that health is normality, since the terms are interchangeable in clinical contexts. But this remark provides no analysis of health until one specifies the norms involved. The most obvious proposal, that they are pure statistical means, is widely recognized to be erroneous. On the one hand, many deviations from the average—e.g. unusual strength or vital capacity or eye color—are not unhealthy. On the other hand, practically everyone has some disease or other, and there are also particular diseases such as tooth decay and minor lung irritation that are nearly universal. Since statistical normality is therefore neither necessary nor sufficient for clinical normality, most writers take the following view about the norms of health: that they must be determined, in whole or in part, by acts of evaluation. More precisely, the orthodox view is that all judgments of health include value judgments as part of their meaning. To call a condition unhealthy is at least in part to condemn it; hence it is impossible to define health in nonevaluative terms. I shall refer to this orthodox view as *normativism*.

1. Thomas S. Szasz, *The Myth of Mental Illness* (New York, 1961); Antony Flew, *Crime or Disease?* (New York, 1973), pp. 40, 42.

Normativism has many varieties, which are often not clearly distinguished from one another by the clinicians who espouse them. The common feature of healthy conditions may, for example, be held to be either their desirability for the individual or their desirability for society. The gap between these two values is a persistent source of controversy in the mental-health domain. One especially common variety of normativism combines the thesis that health judgments are value judgments with ethical relativism. The resulting view that society is the final authority on what counts as disease is typical of psychiatric texts, as illustrated by the following quotation:

> While professionals have a major voice in influencing the judgment of society, it is the collective judgment of the larger social group that determines whether its members are to be viewed as sick or criminal, eccentric or immoral.[2]

For the most part my arguments against normativism will apply to all versions indiscriminately. It will, however, be useful to make a minimal division of normativist positions into strong and weak. Strong normativism will be the view that health judgments are pure evaluations without descriptive meaning; weak normativism allows such judgments a descriptive as well as a normative component.[3]

As an example of a virtually explicit statement of strong normativism by a clinician, consider Dr. Judd Marmor's remark in a recent psychiatric symposium on homosexuality:

> . . . to call homosexuality the result of disturbed sexual development really says nothing other than that you disapprove of the outcome of that development.[4]

If we may substitute "unhealthy" for "disturbed," Marmor is claiming that to call a condition unhealthy is *only* to express disapproval of it. In other words—to collapse a few ethical distinctions—for a condition

2. Ian Gregory, *Fundamentals of Psychiatry* (Philadelphia, 1968), p. 32.

3. R. M. Hare, in *Freedom and Reason* (New York, 1963), chap. 2, argues that no terms have prescriptive meaning alone. If this view is accepted, the difference between strong and weak normativism concerns the question of whether "healthy" is "primarily" or "secondarily" evaluative.

4. Judd Marmor, "Homosexuality and Cultural Value Systems," *American Journal of Psychiatry* 130 (1973): 1208.

to be unhealthy it is necessary and sufficient that it be bad. Now at least half of this view, the sufficiency claim, is demonstrably false of physiological medicine. It is undesirable to be moderately ugly or, for that matter, to lack the manual dexterity of Liszt, but neither of these conditions is a disease. In fact, there are undesirable conditions regularly corrected by physicians which are not diseases: Jewish nose, sagging breasts, adolescent fertility, and unwanted pregnancies are only a few of many examples. Thus strong normativism is an erroneous account of health judgments in their paradigm area of application, and its influence upon mental-health theorists is regrettable.

Unlike Marmor, however, many clinical writers take positions that can be construed as committing them merely to weak normativism. A good example is Dr. Marie Jahoda, who concludes her survey of current criteria of psychological health with these words:

> Actually, the discussion of the psychological meaning of various criteria could proceed without concern for value premises. Only as one calls these psychological phenomena "mental health" does the problem of values arise in full force. By this label, one asserts that these psychological attributes are "good." And, inevitably, the question is raised: Good for what? Good in terms of middle class ethics? Good for democracy? For the continuation of the social *status quo*? For the individual's happiness? For mankind? . . . For the encouragement of genius or of mediocrity and conformity? The list could be continued.[5]

Jahoda may here mean to claim only that calling a condition healthy *involves* calling it good. Her remarks are at least consistent with the weak normativist thesis that healthy conditions are good conditions which satisfy some further descriptive property as well. On this view, "healthy" is a mixed normative-descriptive term of the same sort as "honest" and "courageous." The following passage by Dr. F. C. Redlich is likewise consistent with the weak view:

5. Marie Jahoda, *Current Concepts of Positive Mental Health* (New York, 1958), pp. 76–77. See also her remark in *Interrelations Between the Social Environment and Psychiatric Disorders* (New York, 1953), p. 142: ". . . inevitably at some place there is a value judgment involved. I think that mental health or mental sickness cannot be conceived of without reference to some basic value."

> Most propositions about normal behavior refer implicitly or explicitly to ideal behavior. Deviations from the ideal obviously are fraught with value judgments; actually, all propositions on normality contain value statements in various degrees.[6]

Redlich's term "contain" suggests that he too sees the goodness of something as merely one necessary condition of its healthiness, and similarly for badness and unhealthiness.

Yet even weak normativism runs into counterexamples within physiological medicine. It is obvious that a disease may be on balance desirable, as with the flat feet of a draftee or the mild infection produced by inoculation. It might be suggested in response that diseases must at any rate be prima facie undesirable. The trouble with this suggestion is that it is obscure. Consider the case of a disease that has infertility as its sole important effect. In what sense is infertility prima facie undesirable? Considered in abstraction from the actual effects of reproduction on human beings, it is hard to see how infertility is either desirable or undesirable. Possibly those who see it as "prima facie" undesirable assume that most people want to be able to have more children. But the corollary of this position will be that writers of medical texts must do an empirical survey of human preferences to be sure that a condition is a disease. No such considerations seem to enter into human physiological research, any more than they do into standard biological studies of the diseases of plants and animals. Here indeed is another difficulty for any normativist, weak or strong. It seems clear that one may speak of diseases in plants and animals without judging the conditions in question undesirable. Biologists who study the diseases of fruit flies or sharks need not assume that their health is a good thing for us. On the other hand, there is not much sense in talking about the best interests of, say, a begonia. So it seems that normativists must interpret health judgments about plants and lower animals as analogical, in the same way as would be statements about the courage or considerateness of wolves and rats.

If normativism about health is at once so influential and so objectionable, one must ask what persuasive arguments there are in its

6. F. C. Redlich, "The Concept of Normality," *American Journal of Psychotherapy* 6 (1952): 553.

support. I know of only three arguments, of which one will be treated in the next section. A germ of an argument appears in the passage by Redlich just quoted. Health judgments involve a comparison to an ideal; hence, Redlich concludes, they are "fraught with value judgments." It seems evident, however, that Redlich is thinking of ideals such as beauty and holiness rather than the chemist's ideal gas or Weber's ideal bureaucrat. The fact that a gas or a bureaucrat deviates from the ideal type is nothing against the gas or the bureaucrat. There are normative and nonnormative ideals, as there are in fact normative and nonnormative norms. The question is which sort health is, and Redlich has here provided no grounds for an answer.

A second and equally incomplete argument for normativism is suggested by the first two chapters of Margolis' *Psychotherapy and Morality*.[7] Margolis argues in his first chapter that psychoanalysts have been mistaken in holding that their therapeutic activities can "escape moral scrutiny" (p. 13). From this he concludes that "it is reasonable to view therapeutic values as forming part of a larger system of moral values" (p. 37), and explicitly endorses normativism. But this inference is a non sequitur. From the fact that the promotion of health is open to moral review, it in no way follows that health judgments are value judgments. Wealth and power are also "values" in the sense that people pursue them in a morally criticizable fashion; neither is a normative concept. The pursuit of any descriptively definable condition, if it has effects on persons, will be open to moral review.

These two arguments, like the health literature generally, do next to nothing to rule out the alternative view that health is a descriptively definable property which is usually valuable. Why, after all, may not health be a concept of the same sort as intelligence, or deductive validity? Though the idea of intelligence is certainly vague, it does not seem to be normative. Intelligence is the ability to perform certain intellectual tasks, and one would expect that these intellectual tasks could be characterized without presupposing their value.[8] Similarly, a

7. Joseph Margolis, *Psychotherapy and Morality* (New York, 1966).

8. Exactly what intellectual abilities are included in intelligence is, of course, unclear and may vary from culture to culture. (See N. J. Block and Gerald Dworkin, "IQ, Heritability and Inequality, Part I," *Philosophy & Public Affairs*

valid argument may, for theoretical purposes, be descriptively defined[9] roughly as one that has a form no instance of which could have true premises and a false conclusion. Intelligence in people and validity in arguments being generally valued, the statement that a person is intelligent or an argument valid does tend to have the force of a recommendation. But this fact is wholly irrelevant to the employment of the terms in theories of intelligence or validity. To insist that evaluation is still part of the very meaning of the terms would be to make an implausible claim to which there are obvious counterexamples. Exactly the same may be true of the concept of health. At any rate, we have already seen some of the counterexamples.

Since the distinction between force and meaning in philosophy of language is in a rather primitive state, it is doubtful that weak normativism about health can be either decisively refuted or decisively established. But I suggest that its current prevalence is largely the result of two quite tractable causes. One is the lack of a plausible descriptive analysis; the other is a confusion between theoretical and practical uses of the health vocabulary. The required descriptive analysis I shall try to sketch in the next section. As for the second cause, one should always remember that a dual commitment to theory and practice is one of the features that distinguish a clinical discipline. Unlike chemists or astronomers, physicians and psychotherapists are professionally engaged in practical judgments about how certain people ought to be treated. It would not be surprising if the terms in which such practical judgments are formulated have normative content. One might contend, for example, that calling a cancer "inoperable" involves the value judgment that the results of operating will be worse than leaving the disease alone. But behind this conceptual framework of medical practice stands an autonomous framework of medical theory, a body of doctrine that describes the functioning of a healthy body, classifies various deviations from such functioning as

---

3, no. 4 [Summer 1974]: 333.) But this does not show that for any particular group of speakers "intelligent" is a normative term, i.e. has positive evaluation as part of its meaning.

9. The contrary view, which might be called normativism about validity, is defended by J. O. Urmson in "Some Questions Concerning Validity," *Revue Internationale de Philosophie* 25 (1953): 217–229.

diseases, predicts their behavior under various forms of treatment, etc. This theoretical corpus looks in every way continuous with theory in biology and the other natural sciences, and I believe it to be value-free.

The difference between the two frameworks emerges most clearly in the distinction between disease and illness. It is disease, the theoretical concept, that applies indifferently to organisms of all species. That is because, as we shall see, it is to be analyzed in biological rather than ethical terms. The point is that illnesses are merely a subclass of diseases, namely, those diseases that have certain normative features reflected in the institutions of medical practice. An illness must be, first, a reasonably *serious* disease with incapacitating effects that make it undesirable. A shaving cut or mild athlete's foot cannot be called an illness, nor could one call in sick on the basis of a single dental cavity, though all these conditions are diseases. Secondly, to call a disease an illness is to view its owner as deserving special treatment and diminished moral accountability. These requirements of "illness" will be discussed in some detail shortly, with particular attention to "mental illness." But they explain at once why the notion of illness does not apply to plants and animals. Where we do not make the appropriate normative judgments or activate the social institutions, no amount of disease will lead us to use the term "ill." Even if the laboratory fruit flies fly in listless circles and expire at our feet, we do not say they succumbed to an illness, and for roughly the same reasons as we decline to give them a proper funeral.

There are, then, two senses of "health." In one sense it is a theoretical notion, the opposite of "disease." In another sense it is a practical or mixed ethical notion, the opposite of "illness."[10] Let us now examine the relation between these two concepts more closely.

II. Disease and Illness

What is the theoretical notion of a disease? An admirable explanation of clinical normality was given thirty years ago by C. Daly King.

10. Thomas Nagel has suggested that the adjective "ill" may have its own special opposite "well." Our thinking about health might be greatly clarified if "wellness" had some currency.

> The normal . . . is objectively, and properly, to be defined as that
> which functions in accordance with its design.[11]

The root idea of this account is that the normal is the natural. The
state of an organism is theoretically healthy, i.e. free of disease, insofar as its mode of functioning conforms to the natural design of that
kind of organism. Philosophers have, of course, grown repugnant to
the idea of natural design since its cooptation by natural-purpose
ethics and the so-called argument from design. It is undeniable that
the term "natural" is often given an evaluative force. Shakespeare as
well as Roman Catholicism is full of such usages, and they survive as
well in the strictures of state legislatures against "unnatural acts." But
it is no part of biological theory to assume that what is natural is
desirable, still less the product of divine artifice. Contemporary biology
employs a version of the idea of natural design that seems ideal for
the analysis of health.

The crucial element in the idea of a biological design is the notion
of a natural function. I have argued elsewhere that a function in the
biologist's sense is nothing but a standard causal contribution to a goal
actually pursued by the organism.[12] Organisms are vast assemblages
of systems and subsystems which, in most members of a species, work
together harmoniously in such a way as to achieve a hierarchy of goals.
Cells are goal-directed toward metabolism, elimination, and mitosis;
the heart is goal-directed toward supplying the rest of the body with
blood; and the whole organism is goal-directed both to particular
activities like eating and moving around and to higher-level goals
such as survival and reproduction. The specifically physiological functions of any component are, I think, its species-typical contributions to
the apical goals of survival and reproduction. But whatever the correct analysis of function statements, there is no doubt that biological
theory is deeply committed to attributing functions to processes in
plants and animals. And the single unifying property of all recognized

11. C. Daly King, "The Meaning of Normal," *Yale Journal of Biology and
Medicine* 17 (1945): 493–494. Most definitions of health in medical dictionaries
include some reference to functions. Almost exactly King's formulation also
appears in Fredrick C. Redlich and Daniel X. Freedman, *The Theory and Practice
of Psychiatry* (New York, 1966), p. 113.

12. "Wright on Functions," *The Philosophical Review* 85 (1976): 70-86.

diseases of plants and animals appears to be this: that they interfere with one or more functions typically performed within members of the species.

The account of health thus suggested is in one sense thoroughly Platonic. The health of an organism consists in the performance by each part of its natural function. And as Plato also saw, one of the most interesting features of the analysis is that it applies without alteration to mental health as long as there are standard mental functions. In another way, however, the classical heritage is misleading, for it seems clear that biological function statements are descriptive rather than normative claims.[13] Physiologists obtain their functional doctrines without at any stage having to answer such questions as, What is the function of a man? or to explicate "a good man" on the analogy of "a good knife." Functions are not attributed in this context to the whole organism at all, but only to its parts, and the functions of a part are its causal contributions to empirically given goals. What goals a type of organism in fact pursues, and by what functions it pursues them, can be decided without considering the value of pursuing them. Consequently health in the theoretical sense is an equally value-free concept. The notion required for an analysis of health is not that of a good man or a good shark, but that of a good specimen of a human being or shark.

All of this amounts to saying that the epistemology King suggested for health judgments is, at bottom, a statistical one. The question therefore arises how the functional account avoids our earlier objections to statistical normality. King did explain how to dissolve one version of the paradox of saying that everyone is unhealthy. Clearly all the members of a species can have some disease or other as long as they do not have the same disease. King somewhat grimly compares the job of extracting an empirical ideal of health from a set of defec-

13. The view that function statements are normative generates the third argument for normativism. It is presented most fully by Margolis in "Illness and Medical Values," *The Philosophy Forum* 8 (1959): 55–76, section II. It is also suggested by Ronald B. de Sousa, "The Politics of Mental Illness," *Inquiry* 15 (1972): 187–201, p. 194, and possibly by Flew as well in *Crime or Disease?* pp. 39–40. I think philosophers of science have made too much progress in giving biological function statements a descriptive analysis for this argument to be very convincing.

tive specimens to the job of reconstructing the Norden bombsight from assorted aerial debris (p. 495). But this answer does not touch universal diseases such as tooth decay. Although King nowhere considers this objection, the natural-design idea nevertheless suggests an answer that I suspect is correct. If what makes a condition a disease is its deviation from the natural functional organization of the species, then in calling tooth decay a disease we are saying that it is not simply in the nature of the species—and we say this because we think of it as mainly due to environmental causes. In general, deficiencies in the functional efficiency of the body are diseases when they are unnatural, and they may be unnatural either by being atypical or by being attributable mainly to the action of a hostile environment. If this explanation is accepted,[14] then the functional account simultaneously avoids the pitfalls of statistical normality and also frees the idea of theoretical health of all normative content.

Theoretical health now turns out to be strictly analogous to the mechanical condition of an artifact. Despite appearances, "perfect mechanical condition" in, say, a 1965 Volkswagen is a descriptive notion. Such an artifact is in perfect mechanical condition when it conforms in all respects to the designer's detailed specifications. Normative interests play a crucial role, of course, in the initial choice of the design. But what the Volkswagen design actually *is* is an empirical matter by the time production begins. Thenceforward a car may be in perfect condition regardless of whether the design is good or bad. If one replaces its stock carburetor with a high-performance part, one may well produce a better car, but one does not produce a Volkswagen in better mechanical condition. Similarly, an automatic camera may function perfectly and take wretched pictures; guided missiles and instruments of torture in perfect mechanical condition may serve execrable ends. Perfect working order is a matter not of the worth of the product but of the conformity of the process to a fixed design. In the case of organisms, of course, the ideal of health must be determined by empirical analysis of the species rather than by the intentions of a designer. But otherwise the parallel seems exact. A person who by

14. For further discussion of environmental injuries and other details of the functional account of health sketched in this section, see my forthcoming essay "Health as a Theoretical Concept," *Philosophy of Science* 44 (1977): 542-73.

mutation acquires a sixth sense, or the ability to regenerate severed limbs, is not thereby healthier than we are. Sixth senses and limb regeneration are not part of the human design, which at any given time, for better or worse, just is what it is.

We have been arguing that health is descriptively definable within medical theory, as intelligence is in psychological theory or validity in logical theory. Nevertheless medical theory is the basis of medical practice, and medical practice unquestioningly presupposes the value of health. We must therefore ask how the functional view explains this presumption that health is desirable.

In the case of physiological health, there are at least two general reasons why the functional normality that defines it is usually worth having. In the first place, most people do want to pursue the goals with respect to which physiological functions are isolated. Not only do we want to survive and reproduce, but we also want to engage in those particular activities, such as eating and sex, by which these goals are typically achieved. In the second place—and this is surely the main reason the value of physical health seems indisputable—physiological functions tend to contribute to all manner of activities neutrally. Whether it is desirable for one's heart to pump, one's stomach to digest, or one's kidneys to eliminate hardly depends at all on what one wants to do. It follows that essentially all serious physiological diseases will satisfy the first requirement of an illness, namely, undesirability for its bearer.

This explanation of the fit between medical theory and medical practice has the virtue of reminding us that health, though an important value, is conceptually a very limited one. Health is not unconditionally worth promoting, nor is what is worth promoting necessarily health. Although mental-health writers are especially prone to ignore these points, even the constitution of the World Health Organization seems to embody a similar confusion:

> Health is a state of complete physical, mental, and social well-being, and not merely the absence of disease or infirmity.[15]

Unless one is to abandon the physiological paradigm altogether, this definition is far too wide. Health is functional normality, and as such

15. Quoted by Flew, *Crime or Disease?* p. 46.

is desirable exactly insofar as it promotes goals one can justify on independent grounds. But there is presumably no intrinsic value in having the functional organization typical of a species if the same goals can be better achieved by other means. A sixth sense, for example, would increase our goal-efficiency without increasing our health; so might the amputation of our legs at the knee and their replacement by a nuclear-powered air-cushion vehicle. Conversely, as we have seen, there is no a priori reason why ordinary diseases cannot contribute to well-being under appropriate circumstances.

In such cases, however, we will be reluctant to describe the person involved as ill, and that is because the term "ill" *does* have a negative evaluation built into it. Here again a comparison between health and other properties will be helpful. Disease and illness are related somewhat as are low intelligence and stupidity, or failure to tell the truth and speaking dishonestly. Sometimes the presumption that intelligence is desirable will fail, as in a discussion of qualifications for a menial job such as washing dishes or assembling auto parts. In such a context a person of low intelligence is unlikely to be described as stupid. Sometimes the presumption that truth should be told will fail, as when the Gestapo inquires about the Jews in your attic. Here the untruthful householder will not be described as speaking dishonestly. And sometimes the presumption that diseases are undesirable will fail, as with alcoholic intoxication or mild rubella intentionally contracted. Here the term "illness" is unlikely to appear despite the presence of disease. One concept of each pair is descriptive; the other adds to the first evaluative content, and so may be withheld where the first applies.

If we supplement this condition of undesirability with two further normative conditions, I believe we have the beginning of a plausible analysis of "illness."

A disease is an *illness* only if it is serious enough to be incapacitating, and therefore is
  (i) undesirable for its bearer;
  (ii) a title to special treatment; and
  (iii) a valid excuse for normally criticizable behavior.

The motivation for condition (ii) needs no explanation. As for (iii), the connection between illness and diminished responsibility has often been argued,[16] and I shall mention here only one suggestive point. Our notion of illness belongs to the ordinary conceptual scheme of persons and their actions, and it was developed to apply to physiological diseases. Consequently the relation between persons and their illnesses is conceived on the model of their relation to their bodies. It has often been observed that physiological processes, e.g. digestion or peristalsis, do not usually count as actions of ours at all. By the same token, we are not usually held responsible for the results of such processes when they go wrong, though we may be blamed for failing to take steps to prevent malfunction at some earlier time. Now if this special relation between persons and their bodies is the reason for connecting disease with nonresponsibility, the connection may break down when diseases of the mind are at stake instead. I shall now argue, in fact, that conditions (i), (ii), and (iii) all present difficulties in the domain of mental health.

III. MENTAL ILLNESS

For the sake of discussion, let us simply assume that the mental conditions usually called pathological are in fact unhealthy by the theoretical standard sketched in the last section. That is, we shall assume both that there are natural mental functions and also that recognized types of psychopathology are unnatural interferences with these functions.[17] Is it reasonable to make a parallel extension of the vocabulary of medical practice by calling these mental diseases mental illnesses? Let us consider each condition on "illness."

Condition (i) was the undesirability of an illness for its bearer. Now there are obstacles to transferring our general arguments that physiological health is desirable to the psychological domain. Mental states are not nearly so neutral to the choice of actions as physiological states are. In particular, to evaluate the desirability of mental health

16. A good discussion of this point and of the undesirability condition (i) is provided by Flew in the extremely illuminating second chapter of *Crime or Disease?* Flew takes these conditions as part of the meaning of "disease" rather than "illness"; but since he seems to be working from the ordinary usage of "disease," there may be no real disagreement here.

17. The plausibility of these two claims is discussed at length in my essay, "What a Theory of Mental Health Should Be," *Journal for the Theory of Social Behaviour* 6 (1976): 61-84.

we can hardly avoid consulting our desires; but in the mental-health context it could be those very desires that are judged unhealthy. From a theoretical standpoint desires must be assigned a motivational function in producing action. Thus our wants may or may not conform to the species design. But if our wants do not conform to the species design, it is not immediately obvious why we should want them to. If there is no good reason to want them to, then we have a disease which is not an illness. It is conceivable that this divergence between the two notions is illustrated by homosexuality. It can hardly be denied that one normal function of sexual desire is to promote reproduction. If one does not have a desire for heterosexual sex, however, the only good reason for wanting to have such a desire seems to be that one would be happier if one did. But this judgment needs to be supported by evidence. The desirability of having species-typical desires is not nearly so obvious on inspection as the desirability of having species-typical physiological functions.

One of the corollaries of this point is that recent debates over homosexuality and other disputable diagnoses usually ignore at least one important issue. Besides asking whether, say, homosexuality is a disease, one should also ask what difference it makes if it is. I have suggested that biological normality is an instrumental rather than an intrinsic good. We always have the right to ask, of normality, what is in it for us that we already desire. If it were possible, then, to maximize intrinsic goods such as happiness, for ourselves and others, with a psyche full of deviant desires and unnatural acts, it is hard to see what practical significance the theoretical judgment of unhealthiness would have. I do not actually have serious doubts that disorders such as neuroses and psychoses diminish human happiness. It is also true that what is desirable for a person need not coincide with what the person wants; though an anorectic may not wish to eat, it is desirable that he or she do so. But we must be clear that requests to justify the value of health in other terms are always in order, and there are reasons to expect that such justification will require more evidence in the psychological domain than in the physiological.

We have been discussing the value of psychological normality for the individual, as dictated by condition (i) on illness, rather than its desirability for society at large. Since clinicians often assume that mental health involves social adjustment, it may be well to point out that the functional account of health shows this too to be a debatable assumption requiring empirical support. Certainly nothing in the mere statement that a person has a mental disease entails that he or she is contributing less to the social order than an arbitrary normal individual. There is no contradiction in calling van Gogh or Blake or Dostoyevsky mentally disturbed while admiring their work, even if they would have been less creative had they been healthier. Conversely, there is no a priori reason to assume that the healthy human personality will be morally worthy or socially acceptable. If Freud and Lorenz are right about the existence of an aggressive drive, there is a large component of the normal psyche that is less than admirable. Whether or not they are right, the suggestion clearly makes sense. Perhaps most psychiatrists would agree anyway that antisocial behavior is to be expected during certain developmental stages, e.g. the so-called anal-sadistic period or adolescence.

It must be conceded that *Homo sapiens* is a social species. Other organisms of this class, such as ants and bees, display elaborate fixed systems of social adaptations, and it would be remarkable if the human design included no standard functions at all promoting socialization. On the basis of the physiological paradigm, however, it is not at all clear that contributions to society can be viewed as requirements of health except when they also contribute to individual survival and reproduction. No matter how this issue is decided, the crucial point remains: the nature and extent of social functions in the human species can be discovered only empirically. Despite the contrary convictions of many clinicians, the concept of mental health itself provides no guarantee that healthy individuals will meet the standards or serve the interests of society at large. If it did, that would be one more reason to question the desirability of health for the individual.

Let us now go on to condition (ii) on a disease which is an illness: that it justify "special treatment" of its owner. It is this condition together with (iii) that gives some plausibility to the many recent attempts to explain mental illness as a "social status" or "role."[18] The

18. An example of this approach is Robert B. Edgerton, "On The 'Recognition' of Mental Illness," in Stanley C. Plog and Robert B. Edgerton, *Changing Perspectives in Mental Illness* (New York, 1969), pp. 49–72.

idea that the "sick role" is a special one is consistent with the statistical normality of having some disease or other. Since illnesses are serious diseases that incapacitate at the level of gross behavior, everyone can be minimally diseased without being ill. In the realm of mental health, however, many psychiatrists suggest the stronger thesis that it is statistically normal to be significantly incapacitated by neurosis.[19] A similar problem may arise on Benedict's famous view that the characteristic personality type of some whole societies is clinically paranoid.[20] A statistically normal condition, according to our analysis, can be a disease only if it can be blamed on the environment. But one might plausibly claim that most or all existing *cultural* environments do injure children, filling their minds with excessive anxiety about sexual pleasure, grotesque role models, absurd prejudices about reality, etc. It is at least possible that some degree of neurosis or psychosis is a nearly universal environmental injury in our species. Only an empirical inquiry into the incidence and etiology of neurosis can show whether this possibility is a reality. If it is, however, one can maintain the idea that serious diseases are illnesses only by abandoning one of the presuppositions of the illness concept: that not everyone can be ill.[21]

The last and clearest difficulty with "mental illness" concerns condition (iii), the role of illness in excusing conduct. We said that the idea that serious diseases excuse conduct derives from the model of

19. Only one example of this suggestion is Dr. Reuben Fine's statement that neurosis afflicts 99 percent of the population. See Fine's "The Goals of Psychoanalysis," in *The Goals of Psychotherapy*, ed. Alvin R. Mahrer (New York, 1967), p. 95. I consider the issue of whether all neurosis can be called unhealthy in the essay cited in note 16.

20. See the descriptions of the Kwakiutl and the Dobu in Ruth Benedict, *Patterns of Culture* (Boston: Houghton Mifflin, 1934).

21. A number of clinicians have seriously suggested that people who are ill can be distinguished from those who are well by their presence in your office. One such author goes as far as to calculate an upper limit on the incidence of mental illness from the number of members in the American Psychiatric Association. On a literal reading, this patient-in-the-office test implies that one could wipe out mental illness once and for all by dissolving the APA and outlawing psychotherapy. But the whole idea seems silly anyway in the face of various studies that indicate that the population at large is, by the ordinary descriptive criteria for mental disorder, no less disturbed than the population of clinical patients.

the relation of agents to their own physiology. Unfortunately the relation of agents to their own psychology is of a much more intimate kind. The puzzle about mental illness is that it seems to be an activity of the very seat of responsibility—the mind and character—and therefore to be beyond all hope of excuse.

This inference is hardly inescapable; there is room for considerable controversy to which I cannot do justice here. Strictly speaking, mental disorders are disturbances of the personality. It is persons, not personalities, who are held responsible for actions, and one central element in the idea of a person is certainly consciousness. This means that there may be some sense in contrasting responsible persons with their mental diseases insofar as these diseases lie outside their conscious personalities. Perhaps from a psychoanalytic standpoint this condition is often met in psychosis and neurosis. The unconscious processes that surface in these disorders seem at first sight more like things that happen within us, e.g. peristalsis, than like things we do. But several points make this classification look oversimplified. Unconscious ideas and wishes are still *our* ideas and wishes in a more compelling sense than movements of the gut are our movements. They may have been conscious at an earlier time or be made conscious in therapy, whereupon it becomes increasingly difficult to disclaim responsibility for them. It seems quite unclear that we are more responsible for many conscious desires and beliefs than for these unconscious ones. Finally, the hope for contrasting responsible people with their mental diseases grows vanishingly dim in the case of a character disorder, where the unhealthy condition seems to be integrated into the conscious personality.

In view of these points and the rest of the discussion, I think we must accept the following conclusion. While conditions (i), (ii), and (iii) apply fairly automatically to serious physical diseases, not one of them should be assumed to apply automatically to serious mental diseases. If the term "mental illness" is to be applied at all, it should probably be restricted to psychoses and disabling neuroses. But even this decision needs more analysis than I have provided in this essay. It seems doubtful that on any construal mental illness will ever be, in the mental-health movement's famous phrase, "just like any other illness."

What are the implications of our discussion for the social issues to which psychiatry is so frequently applied? As far as the criminal law is concerned, our results suggest that psychiatric theory alone should not be expected to define legal responsibility, e.g. in the insanity defense.[22] Although the notion of responsibility is a component of the notion of illness, it belongs not to medical theory but to ethics, and one can fix its boundaries only by rational ethical debate. It seems certain that such a simple responsibility test as that the act of the accused not be "the product of mental disease" is unsatisfactory. No doubt many of us have antisocial tendencies that derive from underlying psychopathology of an ordinary sort. When these tendencies erupt in a parking violation or negligent collision, it hardly seems inhumane or unjust to apply legal sanctions.[23] But this is not surprising, for no psychiatric concept is properly designed to answer moral questions. I am not saying that psychiatry is irrelevant to law and ethics. Anyone writing or applying a criminal code is certainly well advised to obtain the best available information about human nature, including the information about human nature that constitutes mental-health theory. The point is that one cannot expect to substitute psychiatry for moral debate, any more than moral evaluations can be substituted for psychiatric theory. Insofar as the psychiatric turn consists in such substitutions, it is fundamentally misconceived.

The other main implications of our discussion seem to me twofold. First, there is not the slightest warrant for the recurrent fantasy that what society or its professionals disapprove of is ipso facto unhealthy. This is not merely because society may disapprove of the wrong things. Even if ethical relativism were true, society still could not fix the functional organization of the members of a species. For this reason it could never be an infallible authority either on disease or on illness, which is a subclass of disease. Thus one main source of the

22. The same conclusion is defended by Herbert Fingarette in "Insanity and Responsibility," *Inquiry* 15 (1972): 6–29.

23. Thus I disagree with H.L.A. Hart, among others, who writes: ". . . the contention that it is fair or just to punish those who have broken the law must be absurd if the crime is merely a manifestation of a disease." The quotation is from "Murder and the Principles of Punishment: England and the United States," reprinted in *Moral Problems*, ed. James Rachels (New York, 1975), p. 274.

tendency to call radical activists, bohemians, feminists, and other unpopular deviants "sick" is nothing but a conceptual confusion.

The second moral suggested by our discussion is that it is always worth asking, in any particular case, how strong the presumption is that health is desirable. When the value of health is left both unquestioned and obscure, it has a tendency to undergo inflation. The diagnosis especially of a "mental illness" is then likely to become an amorphous and peculiarly repellent stigma to be removed at any cost. The use of muscle-paralyzing drugs to compel prisoners to participate in "group therapy" is a particularly gruesome example of this sort of thinking.[24] But there are many other situations in which everyone would profit by asking what exactly is wrong with being unhealthy. In a way liberal reformers tend to make the opposite mistake: in their zeal to remove the stigma of disease from conditions such as homosexuality, they wholly discount the possibility that these conditions, like most diseases, are somewhat unideal. If the value of health, as I have argued in this essay, is nothing but the value of conformity to a generally excellent species design, then by recognizing that fact we may improve both the clarity and the humanity of our social discourse.

24. For this and other "therapeutic" abuses in our prison system, see Jessica Mitford, *Kind and Usual Punishment* (New York, 1973), chap. 8.

LAWRENCE C. BECKER   Human Being:
The Boundaries
of the Concept

I. PROBLEMS OF DEFINITION

Uncertainty about our ability to define the biological boundaries of human life is familiar. Currently, the most prominent issue is the definition of death—specifically whether to retain the traditional cardiopulmonary criteria for death or to adopt some version of so-called brain-death criteria. The law in some jurisdictions has already begun to permit physicians to pronounce death on a finding of "irreversible coma." And though it is clear that transplant surgery and the development of life-support technology have given impetus to the change, a number of writers have taken pains to argue that it is perfectly sound, conceptually, to redefine death.

Problems with the definition of the beginning of human life are even more frequently rehearsed. There are advocates of the biological life-cycle account, various developmental views, theological ensoulment theories, and "personhood" definitions. The United States Supreme Court has recently accepted the view that no conclusive reasons can be found for settling on any one of these rather than another.

The importance of these definitional questions for moral philosophy is obvious. Human beings protect themselves with a thicket of rights they do not grant to other beings, and some of these rights are said to

Earlier versions of this paper were read to the Conference on Moral Problems in Medicine, sponsored by the Council for Philosophical Studies, and to the Philosophy Club of the University of Virginia. Thanks are due to members of both groups for helpful comments, but my particular gratitude extends to Jean W. Hitzeman, James E. Kennedy, Marvin Kohl, and George M. Brockway, who saved me from some serious errors.

be *human* rights—rights one has simply by virtue of being human. Any conceptual uncertainty about when an entity has become or has ceased to be human is a problem for the ascription of such rights. Further, what might be called threshold homicides—the killing of entities whose claim to being human is somewhat in doubt—have become increasingly problematic. There are intraspecies threshold questions (abortion, infanticide, some types of euthanasia) and interspecies threshold questions (the killing of other intelligent life forms).

I am concerned, here, with two propositions about the boundaries of human life, each of which has a direct bearing on current controversies and perennial moral problems:

(1) That there is no decisive way to define, in purely biological terms, either the point at which a human life begins, or the point at which it ends.

(2) In any case, if the end points are going to be used as moral divides, they should be defined in terms of morally relevant characteristics, not purely biological ones.

My purpose is to attack both of these propositions by proposing what I take to be decisive biological definitions of the boundaries and by giving reasons for thinking that, for moral theory, such biological definitions are preferable to "morally relevant" ones. The arguments on the latter issue are fairly straightforward and need not be abstracted in this introduction. But the arguments for the boundary definitions are a bit tortuous, so it may be worthwhile to give an overview of them.

The line of argument for the becoming/being boundary may be summarized as follows:

(1) Entry into the class of human beings is a process.

(2) The entry process is at least in part a biological one.

(3) The completion of the biological part of the entry process is a necessary condition for the completion of the entry process per se.

(4) The biological part of the entry process is developmental in nature—the development of a set of living cells into a multicellular organism.

(5) The developmental nature of the biological part of the entry process is best understood by way of an analogy with metamorphosis—that is, as the genesis, from the relatively undifferentiated mass of the fertilized ovum, of the fundamental morphology and histologically differentiated organs the organism is genetically programmed to develop.

(6) The completion of what I shall call the metamorphic phase of generative development is a necessary condition of the completion of the entry process—that is, the becoming/being boundary cannot be put any earlier than this.

(7) There are no good reasons for putting the boundary any later than this.

(8) Therefore, the becoming/being boundary lies at the completion of the metamorphic phase of generative development.

The line of argument for the being/has-been boundary is parallel:

(1) Exit from the class of human beings is a process.

(2) The exit process is at least in part a biological one.

(3) The completion of the biological part of the exit process is a necessary condition for the completion of the exit process per se.

(4) The biological part of the exit process is disintegrative in nature.

(5) The disintegrative nature of the biological part of the exit process is best construed as the functional disintegration of the organism as such—and not as the physical disintegration of its parts.

(6) The completion of the disintegration of the organism as such is a necessary condition for the completion of the exit process— that is, the being/has-been boundary cannot be put any earlier than this.

(7) There are no good reasons for putting the boundary any later than this.

(8) Therefore, the being/has-been boundary lies at the completion of the disintegration of the human being considered as a biological organism.

Without further ado, then, I shall turn to the arguments for the becoming/being boundary.

II. THE BECOMING/BEING BOUNDARY

A caterpillar is not a butterfly. That is, the insect of which the caterpillar is the larval stage is not, at the larval stage, a butterfly—though one might, as indeed biologists do, speak of butterflies as "adult butterflies" in order to emphasize the fact that both caterpillars and butterflies are stages in the development of the same insect. Nonetheless we do not confuse insects which *are* butterflies with insects of the same species which *are* caterpillars. The latter are *becoming* butterflies no doubt, but they are not butterflies yet.

When can we say that the insect *is* a butterfly as opposed to a caterpillar (or rather, a pupa)? Surely we can say this only when the process of metamorphosis is complete—that is, when the relatively undifferentiated mass left by the disintegration of the caterpillar's tissues has metamorphosed into the pattern of differentiation we call a butterfly.

Human fetal development is a process analogous to metamorphosis, and just as it makes good sense to speak of butterfly eggs, larvae, and pupae as distinct from the butterflies they become (to say that they are *not* butterflies) so too it makes sense to say that human eggs, embryos, and fetuses are distinct from the humans they become—that they are not human *beings*, only human becomings.

When can we say that the fetus is a human being rather than a human becoming? Surely only when its metamorphic-like process is complete—that is, when the relatively undifferentiated mass of the fertilized human ovum has developed into the pattern of differentiation characteristic of the organism it is genetically programmed to become.

That is the core of what I have to say about the becoming/being boundary. But it will require considerable elaboration and defense, and it may help to note, to begin with, that the definitional problem here is to clearly describe a concept of "being"—a static, or at any rate reasonably stable, "completed" condition. This is not to say, of course, that human beings are themselves static or unchanging. It is merely to indicate that we are looking for the boundaries which define membership in the class of living humans—and which distinguish that class from the class of entities which might, but have not yet, become humans, as well as from the class of entities which have been, but are no longer, humans. In the case of the becoming/being boundary, then, we are looking for a point at which the entity is in some very fundamental sense "completed" as a member of the species. I shall argue in what follows that this point is reached when the organism (assumed, of course, to be living) has assumed its basic morphology, and when its inventory of histologically differentiated organs is complete. (It may be worth pointing out one subtlety here. I will argue that the process is complete for a given organism when *that* organism's inventory of organs is complete—not when some standard list of human organs is filled. This is done to account for mutants.)

The rationale for this point as the becoming/being boundary begins with the straightforward observation that entry into the class of living human beings is a process. The claim that "entry is a process" means no more than that humans come into being *by way* of a process. This process is, at least in part, a biological one—involving at a minimum the production of an ovum in a suitable environment for parthenogenesis or cloning, and typically the production of both ovum and sperm, together with the processes necessary for their union. Whatever else we may want to say about this process of entry, we have to concede, surely, that the completion of its biological aspects is a necessary condition of its completion per se. (Whether it is also a sufficient condition will be discussed later.) Thus it is clear that the becoming/being boundary cannot be put at a point prior to the biological completion of the process of entry.

The starting point of the process is not in dispute here, though to put it at conception would beg an important question. So assume that the process starts well before conception—say, with the production of the particular ovum which is to be fertilized (or perhaps "activated" in the case of cloning). The question to be answered, then, is: At what point do we have adequate reasons for saying that the process is biologically complete?

A standard answer is derived from the concept of a "life cycle." The argument is that the life cycle of a human being begins at conception—

just as the life cycle of a butterfly begins with a fertilized egg, progresses through the larval and pupal stages, and culminates in the development of what is popularly described as a butterfly. The trouble with the caterpillar/butterfly analogy as proposed above—according to the life-cycle argument—is that it misleads one into thinking that entry into the *species* coincides with the end of metamorphosis. Quite the contrary: egg, larva, pupa, and butterfly are all stages in the development of *one* entity of *one* species; just as conceptus, embryo, fetus, neonate, infant, child, adolescent, and adult are all stages in the development of one entity of the species *homo sapiens*. "Being" a human thus begins at conception—at the beginning of the life cycle.

This is a rhetorically persuasive argument, but it contains both logical and empirical errors. The fundamental logical error can be seen most clearly by first considering the obviously fallacious syllogism (all too frequently taken seriously):

This conceptus is a being (i.e. is an entity and is alive).
It is certainly human (i.e. is of no other species).

Therefore, it is a human being.

The fallacy here is equivocation on the word "human." As used in the premise it is an adjective—and as such applies not only to the conceptus but to any living part of a member of the species: human blood; human sperm. But as used in the conclusion, "human" functions as a noun meaning "member of the species *homo sapiens*." A counterexample will suffice to make the point.

This sperm cell is a being (i.e. an entity and alive).
It is certainly human (i.e. is of no other species).

Therefore, it is a human being.

The fallacy in the life-cycle argument is not quite as blatant, but it is similar. From the premise that fertilization of the ovum produces a unique living entity which is a product of the species, it does *not* follow that that entity is a *member* of the species. It is just as possible to conclude that the entity produced by fertilization is one which will *become* a member of the species.

The empirical error in the life-cycle definition utterly destroys its plausibility as an account of the becoming/being boundary. Monozy-

gotic twinning can occur any time from the two-cell stage to about
the fourteenth day after conception. And it is thought that most such
twinning is not genetically determined.[1] What this means is that one
cannot say at conception, even given complete knowledge of the
genetic makeup of the conceptus, how many humans will develop
from it. It surely will not do, therefore, to say that the process of becoming *a* human being ends at conception.[2]

But if not at conception, then when? Shall we say that the be-
coming/being boundary lies at the point where the number of embryos is irrevocably determined? Shall we say that the life cycle of a
human being begins at that point? I think not—this time for purely
conceptual reasons.

It has already been noted that there is no logical necessity in the
inference from the premise that a unique, living, and human entity
exists to the conclusion that that entity is a human being—i.e. a
member of the species as opposed to an entity in the process of becoming one. So we are certainly not *forced* to put the boundary at
the end of the twinning possibility. Indeed, I suggest that when we
reflect on the nature of human development, the only point for the
becoming/being boundary which makes conceptual sense is at the
end of what might be called its metamorphic phase. Some detail will
be helpful at this point.

1. See M.G. Bulmer, *The Biology of Twinning in Man* (Oxford, 1970), and
relevant passages from Max Levitan and Ashley Montagu, *Textbook of Human
Genetics* (New York, 1971). The importance of the issue of twinning was
brought to my attention by James M. Humber's paper, "The Immorality of
Abortion," presented at the Eastern Division Meetings of the American Philosophical Association in December 1973. It should be noted, however, that at least
in terms of the arguments of that paper, Mr. Humber would apparently not agree
that this problem is a significant one for the conception definition.

2. One can, of course, assert the contrary by saying that once conception
occurs, nonbiological souls come into being, and that the number of souls thus
brought into being determines (or corresponds to) the number of fetuses which
will develop. One would then have to go on to identify the existence of the
souls with the existence of human beings. But one can assert the contrary of any
proposition whatsoever in this way—assuming the assertion is not self-con-
tradictory. That is, one can merely invent an alternative. The question is, what
reasons can be offered to support the truth of such an alternative claim? I shall
assume here—and it is surely not an arbitrary assumption—that no philosophical-
ly defensible reasons can be found to support the "nonbiological soul" alternative in this context.

"Biological development" is a very broadly defined term. One writer says: "Development may be defined as the action of genes in: (1) creating a new organism from some part of a parent organism, (2) maintaining or increasing the size of a fully formed mature organism, and (3) repairing accidental defects or losses in an organism. . . ."[3] It is clear that the first category above is the sort of development of concern to us here. Let us call it (human) *generative* development, to distinguish it from the other sorts, which are typically referred to as continuous development and regenerative development, respectively.

Human generative development involves four sorts of processes: (a) cell proliferation, in which the number of cells increases; (b) growth, in which there is an increase in the mass of the developing organism; (c) morphogenesis, in which progressive changes in form take place; and (d) histogenesis, in which cells specialize into tissues. Morphogenesis and histogenesis are often lumped together under the title *differentiation*.

Differentiation, cell proliferation, and growth are all involved in continuous and regenerative development as well as in generative development, of course. The continuous production of red blood cells throughout life is an example of histogenesis. Obviously, to speak of the sort of completion indicated by the becoming/being boundary is not to speak of the completion of such processes of maintenance and regeneration—however similar they are in kind to the processes of generative development. It is rather (at least in part) to speak of the completion of the process of the generation of a new (human) organism.

But what is the nature of this process, and when is it complete? While the distinction between the generation, maintenance, and regeneration of an organism is reasonably clear at the most abstract level, how is one to give it application in the case of human development? It is here that the analogy to metamorphosis is helpful.

In common biological usage, "metamorphosis" doubtless refers to the sort of transformations undergone by the developing butterfly—where there is first the generation of a free-living larval body distinctly different from the adult, then the de-differentiation of the tissues of

3. Nelson T. Spratt, Jr., *Developmental Biology* (Belmont, Calif., 1971), p. 5.

that body and the subsequent generation of the adult. But biologists who have addressed themselves to examining the nature of this process characterize it in a way which, without strain, fits human fetal development. Embryonic and metamorphic development are often spoken of conjointly.[4] In fact, as one writer classifies types of metamorphosis, a distinct larval body is not required at all—and thus human generative development sits comfortably as a *type* of metamorphosis.[5]

Now it is clear that generative development has both what might be called *fundamental* aspects and aspects which are essentially refinements of or maturation of the basic structures of the organism. The neonate has a skeletal system of about 270 bones. "Fusion of some of these in infancy reduces this number slightly, but from then until puberty there is a steady increase . . . at puberty there are 350 separate bony masses, and this number is increased still further during adolescence. Thereafter, fusions again bring about a reduction to the final quota of 206. . . ."[6] Similarly with gametogenesis. Oögonia in the female and spermatogonia in the male are present before birth, but their maturation into full-fledged ova (i.e. oötids) and spermatozoa only comes about at puberty. In the case of the lungs, the alveolar ducts are present in the fetus, but only after birth do the alveoli proper develop, and continue to proliferate well into the eighth year of childhood.[7] Examples of such refinement and maturation of structures—undeniably a part of generative development—could be multiplied.

But the original analogy to metamorphosis is instructive here. Just as it is not the size of the entity, or whether its cells are proliferating,

4. Ibid., p. 17; and the following: "Metamorphosis is a widespread developmental phenomenon which is usually associated with a dramatic change in habitat and consequent way of life. . . . Primarily it consists of the differential destruction of certain tissues, accompanied by an increase in growth and differentiation of other tissues. The phenomenon of regional growth and differentiation associated with local cell death in developing limbs comes into this category." N. J. Berrill, *Developmental Biology* (New York, 1971), pp. 423–424.

5. Spratt, *Developmental Biology*, pp. 283–284, quoting Weiss, *The Science of Zoölogy* (New York, 1966).

6. L.B. Arey, *Developmental Anatomy*, 7th ed. (Philadelphia, 1965), p. 405.

7. See J.B. Thomas, *Introduction to Human Embryology* (Philadelphia, 1968), p. 297.

which is at stake in our judgment that the pupa has become a butterfly, so too we are not concerned with various refinements, adaptations to environment outside the cocoon, and maturation which might take place in the butterfly's basic structure. Metamorphosis—*at least in the sense relevant to drawing the line between pupa and butterfly*—is complete once these basic structures are complete. Similarly for humans. Generative development in the form of refinements, adaptations, and maturation of the basic structures are not of concern in drawing the becoming/being boundary.

But what counts as the "basic structure" and when is its generation complete? This is probably a more difficult question empirically than it is conceptually. Conceptually, the answer is not hard to find. The metamorphic phase of generative development (i.e. the "fundamental" differentiation) is complete when (1) the organism has assumed its basic gross anatomical form, normal or not (by which I mean its basic skeletal structure, musculature, arrangement of organ masses, and distribution of tissues); (2) the organism's inventory (normal or not) of histologically differentiated organs is complete.

This is not, notice, a functional criterion so much as an anatomical one. That the developing embryo is "alive"—i.e. functioning as a biological organism—is assumed. The question is when, in the course of its development, we may say that its fundamental or metamorphic generative development is at an end.

It seems indisputable that the end cannot be put any earlier than the point described above. After all, if anything is basic to human generative development (beyond conception) it is the shaping of the formless mass of cells into the shape and general arrangement of parts which the continuous and regenerative processes of development will maintain. And an "organ" which is not histologically differentiated is no organ at all. I do not think anyone would want to hold that the generation of organs was not a part of basic generative development. So the boundary can surely not be put any earlier than the point I have described. And to put the point later than that—to require, for example, that the differentiation of the ciliary muscles of the eye be complete—stretches the notion of fundamental or basic structures beyond reasonable bounds. I do not mean to claim that the distinction between basic and nonbasic generative development is conceptually crisp—such that, given any example of generative development, it could be unarguably classified in one and only one of the categories. I merely hold—and will argue below—that the distinction is clear enough for the use we need to make of it.

The empirical question, however, may be more difficult—or at least it seems so to a nonbiologist reading the standard sources. The completion of gross anatomical form is not much of a problem. That is virtually complete by the end of the third lunar month of gestation—so much so that aborted fetuses of that age can be used in place of cadavers to teach anatomy to medical students. ". . . [W]ith the aid of a simple magnifier, every gross anatomical detail can be seen."[8] Further changes in morphology (e.g. as late as those occurring during puberty) are either the regional growth of existing structures, or clearly in the category of refinements, adaptation, and maturation of those structures.

The histogenesis of organs is a more difficult matter. It is clear that very few organs are histologically differentiated at the end of the third lunar month. Indeed, development of the alveolar ducts and the formation of elastic tissue in the lungs occurs well into the sixth lunar month.[9] Parts of the digestive system (e.g. esophageal glands) are defined even later.[10] The timetable for these later developments is not terribly precise, and no doubt can never be, due to individual variations. But it seems true to say that the end of what I am calling the metamorphic phase of generative development can be put no earlier than the middle of the sixth lunar month of gestation and need not be put any later than the middle of the final month—generative development thereafter clearly falling into the refinement, adaptation, and maturation category. (The various skeletal rearrangements,

8. Hans Elias, *Basic Human Anatomy as Seen in the Fetus* (St. Louis, 1971), p. vii.

9. "Primary ossification centers of the pharyngeal arches appear . . . the circular ciliary muscles of the eye are differentiating. . . . The lumina of parotid and sublingual glands are established . . . primordia of Peyer's patches appear in the ileum. . . . Development of the alveolar ducts including the formation of elastic tissue is prominent. . . . The hyaloid artery of the eye begins to degenerate." J.B. Thomas, *Human Embryology*, pp. 280–281.

10. Ibid., p. 297.

the myelization of neural tissue, the proliferation of alveoli, and gametogenesis are all clearly in the nonbasic category.)

Suppose, then, just for the argument, that we say that the metamorphic phase of generative development is complete at the beginning of the eighth month. Are we then in a position to defend the claim that such a fetus is a human *being* as opposed to a human becoming? Reasons have been given for the contention that the becoming/being boundary cannot be put any earlier than this—that is, that the completion of generative metamorphosis is a necessary condition for entry into the class of human beings. But is it also a sufficient condition? Are there good reasons for thinking that the completion of the metamorphic phase of generative development is enough to count as crossing the becoming/being boundary? I think there are good reasons—conclusive ones in fact—but they are of a negative sort. That is, I think the reasons consist in there being no good reasons for requiring anything further by way of a condition. The clearest way to show this is by dealing with some obvious objections to the metamorphic definition as here proposed.

III. OBJECTIONS TO THE METAMORPHIC DEFINITION

Imprecision

It may be argued that the obvious imprecision in the timetable of metamorphosis is intolerable, as one cannot know in advance—at various points in the last few months of gestation—whether, for example, a particular abortion will be homicide or not.

The reply to this objection may be brief. We are faced with many such uncertainties in both the law and morality. Often we have to deal with a process and need to know precisely when it was "complete," but find the difficulties nearly insuperable. Consider the notorious difficulties of distinguishing an attempted crime (an indictable offense) from the mere preparation to attempt it (which is not an indictable offense).[11] Such problems cannot be solved, they can only

11. See, for example, a standard hornbook on the substantive criminal law: Wayne R. LaFave and Austin W. Scott, Jr., *Handbook on Criminal Law* (St. Paul, 1972), pp. 431–438. For a review of some of the cases and comment on the

be handled. And in the case of the definition of "human being," *if it is to figure in the administration of a stringent prohibition of homicide*, it seems reasonable to adopt an empirically conservative presumption. If basic, generative differentiation has ever been known to be (or can reasonably be thought to have been) complete by the end of the first week of month seven, then one might invoke the presumption of homicide for the destruction of any fetus reasonably believed to be in or beyond the seventh month of gestation. Or one might want to adopt a series of increasingly strong standards of care, beginning at the latest point at which the process can be guaranteed to be incomplete.[12] In any case this is a practical problem of a sort endemic to law and morality, and it is safe to say that the leading alternative candidates for the becoming/being distinction (i.e. conception, viability, and the development of personality) are also subject to it. It cannot, therefore, constitute any special objection to the metamorphic definition.

Mutation and Arrested Development

A critic may want to know more, however, about how the definition handles cases of mutation and arrested development. What about the fetus which develops no limbs, or only one kidney, or a heart with only three valves?

Here it helps to remember that the metamorphic definition—beyond requiring genetic material from the species—is phrased in terms of the development of each individual. Whether that individual has a genetic anomaly which causes a mutation in form or organ inventory, or whether environmental factors put a premature end to development is irrelevant. If the fetus (mutant or not) dies or is killed before the completion of the metamorphic phase of *its* generative development, then what has died or been killed is a human becoming. If the fetus survives, and the process of differentiation is complete, yet the fetus is not normally formed, then what lives is a non-normally formed

---

philosophical aspects of the problem, see my article, "Criminal Attempt and the Theory of the Law of Crimes," *Philosophy & Public Affairs* 3, no. 3 (Spring 1974): 262–294.

12. The Supreme Court has done something similar in its recent abortion decision. See Roe v. Wade 410 U.S. 113, 41 LW 4213 (1973) at 4214.

human being. If the fetus is born prior to the completion of the process, but given the proper environment, can survive while the process continues to completion, then what has been born is a human becoming. It should be noted that none of this implies, by itself, the existence or nonexistence of specific duties toward such fetuses. The morality of the treatment of fetuses of various sorts and in various stages of development is a matter for further argument. It is no objection to the metamorphic definition to show that it does not settle such matters.

Alternatives to the Metamorphic Definition

The first two objections aside, there may be some remaining feeling that the choice of the metamorphic definition is as arbitrary as several other alternatives. Even if conception and the terminus of the twinning possibility have been ruled out, why not choose the concept of viability—on the grounds, perhaps, that a human being is not a biological parasite, but that the fetus is just that until the point of viability? Or why not choose quickening or live birth or the development of personality? To relieve this dissatisfaction, it will be necessary to say a few words about some of the other standard candidates for the becoming/being boundary.

The viability alternative is unsatisfactory. It confuses a criterion with a definition. Viability is not a *definition* of "human being." One can, after all, have a nonviable (but temporarily alive) human being. Viability is rather, in fact, a rough *criterion* for the completion of the process of metamorphosis. Viability (outside the mother's body and outside mechanical facsimilies of it) coincides—roughly—with the end of basic histogenesis as here described.

Other alternatives to the metamorphic definition have even less plausibility. "Quickening" has nothing to recommend it even initially —unless it is confused with viability. The point of "live birth" is flatly arbitrary, bearing as it does no necessary relation to properties of the fetus. It has some advantages as a legal device for fixing age, but beyond that, has nothing to recommend it.[13] And the development

13. That is, there is nothing to recommend it as a becoming/being boundary. As a moral distinction based on the fact that the neonate immediately begins "to play an explicit role within the social structure of the family and society"

of "personhood," as a definition of human being, only has interest if
one is singlemindedly trying to build up a definition which will yield
"rights to life"—where such rights are understood to arise only from
the claims one agent may make on another. It taxes the concept of
membership in the species too far to say that a fourteen-year-old, so
catastrophically deficient as to warrant the claim that he or she is not
a "person," is not a member of the species.

The Moral Emptiness of the Definition

But then, it may be urged, one has abandoned any attempt to make
the becoming/being boundary a moral divide. One can understand
how quickening might be held to have characteristics relevant to a
moral boundary—for it has a psychological impact on the pregnant
woman and others. Similarly with live birth and the development of
personality. But "the end of the metamorphic phase of generative development" does not seem to capture any morally significant distinction. And the resistance to adopting a morally empty definition, given
our actual use of rough and ready becoming/being boundaries as
moral divides is strong. As Tooley and others have argued, if the
legitimacy of moral prohibitions and permissions (say, with regard
to killing) are going to rest on whether or not the victim has crossed
the becoming/being boundary, then the drawing of that boundary
must be done in terms of characteristics relevant to the moral justification of those prohibitions and permissions.[14] This is an important
line of argument, so I want it to be clear why I reject its applicability
here.

In the first place, I think we may plausibly reject quickening and
live birth as candidates for the sort of moral divide at stake here. We
are, after all, talking about *duties* not to kill, and the sort of psychological pulls created by these two events (aside from the fact that not
every parent will feel them) are just not the sort of grounds advocates
of a morally relevant definition are interested in. They are interested

there may be more to say for it. See H. Tristam Engelhardt, Jr., "The Ontology
of Abortion," *Ethics* 84 (1974): 217–234, especially pp. 230–232.

14. See Michael Tooley, "Abortion and Infanticide," *Philosophy & Public
Affairs* 2, no. 1 (Fall 1972): 37–65.

in justifying a right *in the victim* not to be killed—a so-called right to life.

Now if one tries to derive the moral rules concerning homicide from special rights to life possessed by the victims and wants to show that those rights to life are derived from some characteristics which define the victims as human beings, then the metamorphic definition is indeed beside the point. So, I believe, are all other nontheological definitions except personhood. The question really is, then, why not adopt personhood as the becoming/being boundary? Even if it leads to unpleasant conclusions such as a failure to rule out infanticide, at least it marks a moral divide of major proportions. Persons—more exactly, self-conscious subjects of experience—can value themselves. And in just the same sense in which my values for my act *A* support the rationality of that act *A*, so too another person's values *against* (my act) *A* support the rationality of (my act) *non-A*. Thus there is one clear sense in which persons can make claims on us which nonpersons cannot make. And since the making of such claims has an obvious application to the question of homicide, it is tempting to try to base one's account of the morality of homicide on such claims.

But I think it is not usually recognized just how unsatisfactory this whole approach is. For one thing, though an obviously sound basis for moral argument, it is a very slender reed on which to hang the whole analysis of homicide. To suppose that all our duties not to kill come from the victim's *rights* (to life, liberty, or whatever), and that those rights are grounded in the victim's ability (and title) to claim certain acts and forbearances from others, is to put oneself in a very awkward position theoretically—not to say morally. What account is one to give, then, of a parent's duties to his or her infant offspring? What account is one to give of our duties not to kill the sleeping? Or temporarily comatose? Or our duties to resuscitate those who have drowned? One is forced, on this account, either to deny the existence of such duties or to construct an account of how such duties can arise from counterfactual conditions (i.e. if *B* were awake, or at the age of reason, or alive again, he would lay claim on me for *X*).

Surely either of these positions is implausible. The counterfactual account is an awkward contrivance in many of these cases. But beyond that, both alternatives ignore some obviously sound lines of moral argument which derive duties from considerations which begin with the *agent*, rather than with the one acted upon. A duty not to kill (or a duty to rescue) may be justified by reference to the consequences for the agent or society. It may be justified as an entailment of the agent's role (parent, doctor, friend). Or it may be justified as a requirement of those patterns of life or character traits of which we can justifiably approve, morally. None of these justifications makes essential reference to the victim's ability and title to lay claim to the duty.

Now I am not suggesting that such agent-based approaches can, by themselves, be any more adequate than the victim-based approach. A general account of the morality of killing which ignored the victim's claims on the agent would be indefensibly incomplete. But so is an account which ignores the agent-based approaches. And once the need for both sorts of approaches is recognized, the attempt to rig a definition of "human being" along the lines suggested by *any* single line of argument (whether victim-based or not) seems arbitrary in the extreme. There can, for example, be no a priori guarantee that the range of entities protected by duties generated from agent-based approaches will coincide exactly with those protected by duties generated from victim-based approaches. So at the least it is certainly an invitation to question-begging to force the terms "human being" and "homicide" into the area circumscribed by the victim-based approach.

Further, of course, the question of homicide not only involves threshold problems (i.e. whether the victim is a human being or not). It also involves giving a rationale for retaining or rejecting all the intricacies of homicide law—the grading of various sorts of homicide, the exculpatory claims we recognize, and the category of justifiable homicide. Any "right to life" which could conceivably be encapsulated in a definition of "human being" would prove an infertile ground indeed for these matters. Consider: appeals to personhood are of no avail in explaining the distinctions we draw between deaths produced by tortious negligence, criminal negligence, and premeditated acts of murder. Human victims of each have, one assumes, an equal "right to life," and surely, *with respect only to that right*, no less a claim on their fellows for reasonable care as for nonmalicious conduct.

It is, of course, possible to build up an account of the details of homicide law by reference to other principles, using the "right-to-life" notion merely as a starting point. But then one must acknowledge, surely, that the "right to life" is itself very nearly vacuous, morally. It functions as nothing more than a general presumption against a certain restricted class of morally problematic killings, and even then it is not relevant to deciding many of the questions we need answered about homicide. This, together with the difficulties of even explicating any morally relevant definition of the "point of entry into humanness" shows, I think, that the objection of vacuousness against the metamorphic definition is without much force.

Indeed, I reiterate that the primacy of the right-to-life line of argument is a snare. A much more straightforward, and thus conceptually clear, approach is simply to ask what presumptions against the taking of life there are, and why, and under what conditions those presumptions may be overcome. A consideration of right-claims made by one agent on another will be a part of this approach, but it is clear that the approach will not be limited to such considerations. Presumptions with regard to the taking of all lives (vegetable, animal, human, potential, or actual) will be confronted directly—not through a mystifying (and doubtless largely self-serving) thicket of special rights definitionally borne by human beings.

This approach to the morality of homicide seems to me to offer more hope of productive, reasoned discussion than do the usual arguments. It will not be easy to specify the grounds for or against a strong presumption concerning the homicide of the fetus of eight months as opposed to a weaker presumption, or none at all, against feticide prior to eight months. But at least the need for argument and the general range of relevant considerations will not be obscure. One may want to begin with a consideration of the prohibition of homicide in the case of healthy adult victims. One would ask for the justification of the prohibition and for the justification of the various exculpatory claims we allow (or ought to allow). One would then work out to threshold questions, such as abortion and euthanasia, in stages, asking the same questions for each stage. Such a process would be uncomfortable, because it would call into question one of our most central and deeply felt moral principles. But unless wisdom profits from evasion, this is exactly what needs to be done. The definition of the becoming/being boundary bears no a priori relevance to this sort of investigation. And if there is a cogent biological definition of the boundary—as I have argued there is—there is no point in resisting it for the purposes of moral theory.

IV. THE BEING/HAS-BEEN BOUNDARY

I said at the outset that the definition of "human being" had to separate not only "being" from "becoming" but also "being" from "has been." I want to conclude by deploying an argument to do this—both to complete the promise and to underline my point about the proper approach to the morality of homicide. Given the fervor with which the definition of death is being discussed currently, the brevity of the argument to follow may be perceived as a fault. But I believe that, unlike the becoming/being distinction, the definition of death presents no serious conceptual problems. There are serious empirical problems associated with the clinical determination of when death occurs, and serious moral problems concerning the treatment of the dying and the dead, but those are separate matters. I shall comment on their relation to the definition of death as the argument proceeds.

On the view proposed here a human being is a biological organism, complete as a living "being" of the species when the metamorphic phase of generative development is complete. Death for such an organism is the same as for any other complex organism. It is a process. The process is, at least in part, a biological one. The completion of the biological part of the process is a necessary condition for its completion per se. This much I take as not needing argument.

I further take it that we may plausibly regard organic death as the completion of the biological part of the "exit process." This introduces an apparent asymmetry into the account, for the becoming/being boundary was drawn in terms of structure, not function. But it should be remembered that the organic life of the developing entity was presupposed as a necessary condition of "human-beinghood." It simply was shown not to be a sufficient condition. But just as organic life precedes the generation of the structures necessary for entry into human-beinghood, so too death precedes the physical disintegration of (most of) those structures. Since life is a necessary condition for biological entry into human-beinghood, its removal (death) is sufficient for marking the completion of the biological part of exit from human-beinghood. The exit process, then, in its biological aspects, is to be construed as a loss of function, not structure.

The being/has-been boundary can thus not be put any earlier than the biological death of the organism. And I shall assume that human beings are mortal in such a way that there is no question but that biological death is a *sufficient* condition for marking the being/has-been boundary. I assume, in particular, that consciousness does not persist beyond organic death.

The interesting question is, of course, What counts as the death of a human being considered as a biological organism? Clearly, parts of an organism may die without bringing about the death of the organism as such. Organisms may lose parts (limbs or organs) and continue to function organically. They are not "partially dead" for that reason. They are simply organisms of a certain type without certain parts. Further, organisms may lose functions necessary to their survival. If these functions are provided mechanically, and thus the organism survives as an organism, it is not dead, it is simply an organism kept alive mechanically.

The biological death of a human organism may be quite straightforwardly described: a human organism is dead when, for whatever reason, the system of those reciprocally dependent processes which assimilate oxygen, metabolize food, eliminate wastes, and keep the organism in relative homeostatis are arrested in a way which the organism itself cannot reverse. It is the confluence of these and only these conditions which could possibly define organic death, given the nature of human organic function. Loss of consciousness is not death any more than is the loss of a limb. The human organism may continue to function as an organic system. Further, though the loss of one vital function (say loss of the capacity to eliminate wastes) may inevitably *bring about* death, it does not constitute death by itself. Nor would we even say that an arrest of *all* the vital functions, in such a way that the organism *itself* could "restart" them, was death. (Consider the legal fate of one who maliciously intervened to prevent the "restart." Surely we would regard such a person as a murderer, and we would not be speaking metaphorically. On the other hand, when an organism has failed in such a way that it cannot restart its organic

processes, *but could be resuscitated by someone else*, what would be
the legal fate of one who maliciously refused to resuscitate? Surely
not an indictment for murder.)

Now it may be objected that requiring the confluent cessation of *all*
the organic functions mentioned is too strong. First, they usually do
not cease simultaneously, and second, it would be somewhat strange
to withhold the judgment of death from an organism whose sole remaining organic function was some waning remnant of the digestive
process, such as the action of enzymes in the intestines. True. But
the definition proposed here does not entail such a result. Death is
defined as the conjoint (not necessarily simultaneous) cessation of
the system of those reciprocally dependent processes which assimilate
oxygen, etc. Some of these processes involve the production of bio-
chemical agents (e.g. enzymes) which, as to their continued existence
and operation, are then relatively independent of the processes which
produced them. But the continued action of such agents, in the
absence of the process which produced them, cannot properly be
considered the continuance of the process. It is rather the action of
isolated remnants of a process which has itself disintegrated. There
are many such events which continue as artifacts of vital processes
after death. A cell may live, though the organ of which it is a part is
dead (i.e. no longer functions as an integrated subsystem of an
organism). An organ or tissue may remain functional for days after
the death of the organism as a whole (as with the cornea or blood
removed from the body or skin kept protected from bacteria). None
of these events embarrass the definition of death given here.

It should be emphasized, however, that this definition of death is to
be sharply distinguished from the notion of a clinical criterion for the
death of a given individual. When we may correctly say that an organism has ceased to function as an organism in the requisite sense
is an empirical problem of considerable delicacy. Fortunately for
moral purposes, the functional disintegration of the human organism
(if not mechanically assisted) is marked by reasonably unambiguous
clinical signs whose "appearance" (e.g. the registering of cardiopulmonary failure) takes a relatively short duration. So no one
exercising reasonable care is likely to have to rush the determination.
(Certain emergency situations are, of course, exceptions.)

Where mechanical assistance is provided to maintain organic function, the implications of the definition of the human being/has-been
boundary are fairly clear. One whose heart no longer functions and
who is kept alive by machine is just that—a human being whose heart
does not function. One who, after a massive accident, has a flat electroencephalogram and no spontaneous respiration, heart activity, or
kidney function, and whose organs are bypassed or kept functioning
by heroic medicine is just that. The definition makes no reference to
the "higher" functions characteristic of humans or to how organic
function is maintained. (After all, in the ninth month of gestation, not
very many "higher" functions are going on, and the fetus functions as
an organism partly by virtue of assistance provided by the mother's
body.)

This is, surely, not only a common-sense view, but one which faces
the moral problems raised by heroic medicine and euthanasia directly.
The moral question here is not whether the permanently comatose are
"really human." The question is, Under what circumstances ought one
to use heroic measures on humans who would otherwise die, and once
in use, under what circumstances may they be withdrawn? Similarly
for questions of "positive" euthanasia. Much clarity is lost, I think, by
organizing inquiries into these matters in terms of a definition of
"human being" which settles the issues. Such definitions merely push
the important questions back one notch (or worse, allow people to
evade them), and inevitably seem ad hoc in nature.

Locutions such as "brain death" are thus misleading when construed as definitions of death. Brain death is not a definition of death,
nor even a criterion of death. It is merely a criterion for deciding
when coma is irreversible.[15] The moral question, accurately put, is,
What should be done with human beings who are in irreversible coma?

There is considerable pressure to resist this conclusion and to allow
physicians to pronounce death upon a finding of irreversible coma.[16]

15. The Harvard Medical School panel charged with defining "brain death"
conflates these questions misleadingly. See their report in Henry K. Beecher,
Research and the Individual (Boston, 1970), pp. 311–319.

16. As recommended by the Harvard panel, ibid., and as is beginning to get
legal recognition, both in cases and in statutes. See, for example, the Kansas
statute defining death, reprinted in Jay Katz, *Experimentation with Human*

The motives behind the move are not hard to discern. Beyond a point which can be specified empirically with some accuracy, hope for bringing the patient back to any form of consciousness—no matter how rudimentary—is simply gone. The brain literally liquifies. And even with the most sophisticated mechanical aids, the other vital organs begin a slow but certain course of degeneration. Leaving aside the desire of some for organs suitable for transplantation, it is an enormously expensive and futile effort to keep such hopelessly comatose patients alive.[17] To be able to pronounce them dead would be a great convenience. It would eliminate any legal hazards involved in "pulling the plug" (for if such patients are regarded as living, turning off the respirators or other devices already in use amounts to active, rather than passive, euthanasia—to killing rather than to letting die). There are, in most cases, no legal obligations to begin such treatment (no legal duty to rescue); but there are often moral obligations, because it is often not clear before the efforts are made whether or not the patient is in irreversible coma. The irony is that once treatment is begun, there is often a legal obligation to continue, although there may be no moral obligation to do so.

Rigging the definition of death to solve this problem, while tempting, is an avoidance of the real issue. The real issue is whether and, if so, when it is moral to give up trying to prolong the patient's life. Putting this question in terms of euthanasia or even "letting people die" is a misleading sensationalization of the issue. Euthanasia is certainly an important moral question in its own right, but the typical medical situations—at least the ones in which the temptation to bring in the definition of "human being" arises—are those in which efforts to prolong life are underway, and the question is whether it makes sense to go on with them. "Giving up" is not always irrational or

---

Beings (New York, 1973), p. 1085, and also the discussion of cases, pp. 1076–1077, 1102–1104.

17. For the presentation of a startling argument that we need to pronounce death in these cases precisely so we can *not* pull the plug but repeatedly "harvest" this new sort of corpse—for the blood it continues to produce, as an experimental object, as a training object for medical students, etc., see Willard Gaylin, "Harvesting the Dead," *Harper's*, September 1974, pp. 23–30.

immoral—and certainly not always illegal.[18] It seems best to face this problem directly—by defining when it is permissible to give up life-saving efforts—and not to evade the problem by introducing an ad hoc definition of death.

The being/has-been boundary thus should not be, by itself, a moral divide any more than the becoming/being boundary is. People live, but sometimes in such hopeless conditions that one may morally and legally give up trying to save them. People die, but sometimes can be revived. Their death does not in itself relieve us of moral obligations toward them.[19] The reversibility of death is more likely the

18. It has been argued that what I have called "giving up" should be regarded in law as a nonculpable *omission*. See George P. Fletcher, "Prolonging Life," *Washington Law Review* 42 (1967): 999. It is a persuasive argument.

19. Consider the astonishing case reported by Beecher, *Research and the Individual*, p. 160, n. 8:

A 5-year-old boy, for example, was submerged for 22 minutes in a Norwegian river at a temperature of -10°C. Before he went under, he was seen in the water clinging to the ice. Doubtless his body temperature rapidly fell during this period, and the resulting hypothermic state probably accounts for his survival. Although the boy seemed to be dead, with blue-white skin and widely dilated pupils, he was given mouth-to-mouth insufflation. The mouth and pharynx were filled with vomitus. This was partially cleared. No pulse was felt. The trachea was intubated, the airway aspirated, artificial respiration instituted, and external heart compression started at once and continued on the way to the hospital. On arrival, there was some evidence of peripheral circulation. The ear lobes became pink. The heart was pricked with a needle and epinephrine and procaine were administered, without apparent result. Blood was withdrawn for typing and for determining the extent of hemolysis. Two and one-half hours after submersion, the heart started to contract spontaneously. Chlorpromazine was administered in an effort to improve the peripheral circulation. Gasping breaths now followed and soon became normal, but in an hour pulmonary edema appeared. Lanatoside and theophyllamine and morphine were given to control it. Three more pulmonary edema episodes ensued. An exchange transfusion was given to eliminate the free hemoglobin and potassium. Respiratory failure occurred five times in the next 24 hours. Hydrocortisone, antibiotics, heparin, and chlorpromazine were given. He was transfused. Examination two days after the accident showed no pupillary or corneal reflexes and no reaction to painful stimuli. On the fifth day, these signs returned. In a week, the boy began to swallow and to cough. On the tenth day he could obey simple commands, recognize his mother, and say "Yes," or "No." The next day he began to shriek and became restless and unconscious. Except for the brief period mentioned, he was unconscious for about six weeks. The agitated period lasted 14 days. He seemed to be decerebrated. Gradual improvement followed, but he appeared to be blind. Six weeks

moral divide. But even irreversible death does not (under our ordinary convictions) mean we can do just as we please with what remains— e.g. the estate; the body. The morality of dealing with the dead, whether reversibly dead or not, is a matter for further argument. It is not settled by this definition of death.

Bizarre questions may be raised, of course. Is a human brain separated from its body and kept "functioning" a human being? (Assuming that the removal of limbs or eyes or heart and lungs would still "leave" a human being.) I admit to being at a loss for a reply to such cases, let alone an answer.

But the inability of a definition to settle bizarre cases need not be considered an overwhelming defect. Bizarre cases can often be settled only by equally bizarre definitions. The definitions proposed here —for both the becoming/being and the being/has-been boundaries— make good sense conceptually, are sufficiently clear for moral purposes, and direct our attention to the moral issues surrounding homicide in a productively direct way. That much, it seems to me, is enough to expect from definitions.

To summarize the conclusions, then, from the somewhat tortuous path just trod: I have argued that

(1) There are rationally preferred choices for both the becoming/ being and being/has-been boundaries, drawn in purely biological terms. The former boundary lies at the completion of the metamorphic phase of generative development; the latter at the functional disintegration of the human being considered as a biological organism.

(2) Neither of these boundaries is, by itself, a moral divide.

---

after the accident his mental condition improved. He began to speak, but still seemed to be blind. A week later, his vision began to return. On discharge, two-and-a-half months after the accident, he behaved like a normal child, except for a little ataxia. Six months after the accident, his mental condition was almost normal for his age, although he was still clumsy, and peripheral vision was reduced. Neurologic examination, including an electroencephalogram, was normal. By the usual clinical standards, he behaved as a normal child.

(3) Each of the boundaries is precise enough for use as a moral divide if further argument establishes the legitimacy of it.
(4) Such further argument cannot reasonably be only of the "victim's right-to-life" variety.
(5) As it turns out, on the abortion question, the United States Supreme Court's advocacy of graduated stages of state interest fits the becoming/being boundary reasonably well.
(6) "Brain death" is neither a definition of, nor a criterion for, the being/has-been boundary.

Doubtless other conclusions are implicit in the arguments. For the moment I content myself with these.

MICHAEL B. GREEN &
DANIEL WIKLER

Brain Death and Personal Identity

The legal and medical definition of death has recently changed in many states from cessation of heart and lung function to so-called brain death. Patients who have suffered irreversible loss of brain function but continue to breathe would have been accounted alive under previous medical practice and legal statute. They are now pronounced dead. Though the changes are sanctioned by leading medical and legal authorities, they have proceeded in a climate of some confusion, a symptom of which was a recent ruling by a Florida judge: "This lady is dead and has been dead and she is being kept alive artificially."[1] In part this confusion is merely the result of misunderstanding on the part of judges and the public of what those authorities proposing redefinition have in mind, but it also mirrors the conceptual disarray in the brain-death literature.[2] Though a large number of physicians, jurists, and philosophers now hold that brain death is death, there is little agreement about the justification for the redefinition or about the nature of the task of "redefinition" itself.

1. *New York Times*, 5 December 1976.
2. Though the literature on brain death is large, it has been remarkably free of argument. The medical literature, especially, gives the reader the impression that no argument is needed. (This sentiment is discussed in part I and II below.) The arguments which we seek to refute are our reconstruction of what we believe to be the assumptions of the leading writers on the subject. Our references to that literature will be accordingly sparse. Two appropriately argumentative papers, with which we take special care to note parts of agreement and contrast, appeared in *Philosophy & Public Affairs*: Lawrence Becker's "Human Being: The Boundaries of the Concept," vol. 4, no. 4 (Summer 1975): 334-359 and above, pp. 23-48, and David Lamb's "Diagnosing Death," vol. 7, no. 2 (Winter 1978): 144-153.

The principal arguments for classifying brain-dead patients as dead can be sorted into two groups. Those of the first type, which we will call the biological arguments, hold that redefinition is required by new developments in biomedical science. The second sort of argument proposes the redefinition as a solution to a moral problem, that of indefinitely and pointlessly maintaining the irreversibly comatose, and hence justified on moral grounds. Each kind of argument has an initial persuasiveness, but this is lost when the arguments are set out and examined in detail. We will argue, in Sections I and II, respectively, that neither of these kinds of arguments supports the thesis that brain-dead patients are dead.

In so arguing, we undermine the principal theoretical sources of support for the new definition of death. Our ultimate intention is, however, to support the brain-death definition. To justify it, we provide, in Section III, what we regard as the first satisfactory rationale for regarding brain death as death. Our argument is ontological rather than biological or moral, having to do with the conditions of existence of persons.[3] We sketch what we believe to be the best theory of personal identity and draw a corollary on brain death which supports the view that persons cease to exist at that moment.

Our conclusion, then, is that brain-dead patients are indeed dead, though not for the reasons that they are now thought of as dead. Whether the brain dead should be considered dead *under the law* is, we argue in Section IV, another issue entirely; we think they should, but provide an argument for the legal redefinition which is wholly independent of our philosophical claim.

I. The Biological Arguments

Brain death—the irreversible cessation of brain function—involves two catastrophic changes in functioning. One is coma, the permanent loss of consciousness and awareness of the world. The other is the loss of

3. The notion that brain death marks the "death of the person" is common in writing on brain death, but usually receives little explicit explication or support, deriving instead either from an intuitive essentialism (see Robert Veatch, *Death, Dying and the Biological Revolution: Our Last Quest for Responsibility,* New Haven: Yale University Press, 1976) or moral considerations (see below, Section II). We distinguish these approaches below, see fn. 28.

the brain's ability to regulate certain autonomic body processes, such as respiration, which contribute to maintenance of internal homeostasis. These losses involve cessation of functioning of different parts of the brain (here for convenience to be called "upper" and "lower," respectively—the details do not matter) and each can occur without the other.[4] The early, influential Harvard Report used the title "A Definition of Irreversible Coma," but consisted of instructions on diagnosing cessation of both upper and lower brain functioning, and left the reader unclear as to which event was meant to mark the patient's death.[5] The subsequent medical literature is not unanimous on this point, but the established view now seems to be that brain death is to be understood as cessation of all brain functioning.[6]

This point is widely misunderstood. In the celebrated case of Karen Quinlan, for example, none of the parties to the dispute over termination of care advanced the claim that she was dead or brain dead, even though she was thought to be in a "persistent vegetative state," that is, shorn of mental capacities.[7] It was thus unfortunate that the case was publicized as a test case for the new definition. Ms. Quinlan was (and is, as of this writing) alive according to the dominant medical brain death conception, since her lower brain continued to regulate her breathing and other life processes. Death is marked, on this view, by death of the *whole* brain. Permanent loss of consciousness has no bearing on the matter if the lower brain continues to do its work. Why have most medical authorities thought that loss of this capacity, as occurs in whole brain death, should be counted as death? As we shall

4. We will use the terms "upper" and "lower" to designate the parts of the brain which sponsor cognitive and regulative functions, respectively. These are not terms of the physiologist's art; it is possible that this neat division of brain parts is false to the facts and that some sections of the brain are involved in both kinds of activity, but we do not see how the present discussion would be thereby undermined.

5. *Journal of the American Medical Association* 205 (1968): 337-340.

6. The physiological facts are elegantly summarized in Peter McL. Black, "Brain Death," *New England Journal of Medicine* 299 (17 August 1978): 338-344; and (24 August 1978): 393-401.

7. New Jersey Supreme Court: In the Matter of Karen Quinlan, an alleged incompetent. 79 NJ 10, 355 A2nd 647 (1976). Our analysis of the matter will vindicate common intuition that Karen Quinlan was already dead while what was once her body continued to live.

argue in Section II, most of the support for redefinition derives from moral considerations. Nevertheless, two arguments have appeared which attempt to uphold the redefinition on medical grounds. The first claims that despite appearances, this is nothing more than an application of the traditional definition of death, one which has heretofore been almost universally accepted. The second sees whole brain death as a departure from tradition, but one justified on scientific grounds. We shall present and counter these in turn.

Brain Death as the Traditional Standard

Has brain death been our traditional definition of death? According to *Black's Law Dictionary*, death is "the ceasing to exist; defined . . . as a total stoppage of the circulation of the blood, and a cessation of the animal and vital functions consequent thereon, such as respiration, pulsation, etc." Since a brain-dead patient, with machine assistance, can exhibit all of these vital signs, it would seem that a pronouncement of death on such a patient would be a clear deviation from the old standard. Yet some of those arguing for the redefinition of death deny this.[8] Their argument first makes a distinction between the state of death and the signs or clinical indicators by which the presence of that state is detected. Thus, a switch from a set of cardiovascular indicators to the set of brain-death indicators need not mean that one tests for different states before declaring brain death.[9] Indeed, according to their argument, the traditional heart-lung test has been a test for brain death all along.

The claim that the traditional heart-lung test has always been used

8. This version of the argument is implicit in much of the brain-death literature, but it has not been spelled out in the form given here. Arguments resembling (inexactly) the one given here may be found in Clarence Crafoord, "Cerebral Death and the Transplant Era," *Diseases of the Chest* 55, no. 2 (February 1969): 141-145; and Robert Schwager, "Medicine and Irreversible Coma," in Tom Beauchamp and Seymour Perlin, eds., *Ethical Issues in Death and Dying* (Englewood Cliffs, 1977).

9. For certain practical reasons, some statutes have written brain death into the legal definition of death alongside, rather than in place of, the traditional heart-lung definition. See Alexander M. Capron and Leon R. Kass, "A Statutory Definition of the Standards for Determining Human Death: An Appraisal and a Proposal," *University of Pennsylvania Law Review* 121, no. 1 (November 1972): 87-118.

to detect brain death is to be secured by the following sub-argument. The presence of heartbeat and breathing in the healthy individual is a sign, not only of heart and lung function, but also of a certain underlying *capacity*, in particular the capacity for spontaneous respiration and heartbeat. Call this Capacity S. The state of death is assumed, on this account, to be the loss of this capacity. The presence of heartbeat and breathing is a good indicator of the presence of S under ordinary circumstances. When heartbeat and breathing are occurring as the result of machine maintenance of life-functions, however, the test yields a false positive. The advent of these artificial aids has made development of a more accurate test mandatory. And (the argument continues) this is what the direct tests for brain function are. Capacity S is lodged in the lower brain; use of the EEG and similar indicators of brain death give us a direct reading on the presence of S regardless of clinical context. Hence brain death represents only a technological refinement of the traditional indicators of death, and no change in the definition of death at all.

The troubles with this argument are twofold. First, Capacity S—the capacity for spontaneous heartbeat and respiration—is *not* lodged in the lower brain. If it were, a functional lower brain would guarantee the presence of S. But it does not. If "spontaneous" means unassisted by machine, S is a capacity of the body as a whole. Hence brain death is not the same as loss of Capacity S. Second, loss of Capacity S was not the state tested for by the traditional tests for death. Persons requiring pacemakers because of heart injury, or respirators due to spinal injury, also lack this capacity. But they are surely not to be counted as dead for that reason by the concept of death embodied in the traditional definition. Machine dependence *in general* has no bearing on one's status as alive or dead.[10] But Capacity S involves nothing more than general machine independence: the ability to breathe and to circulate blood without artificial support. But since the absence of S has never been the state of death, it hardly matters that brain death is an unfailing indicator of it. Hence it is no argument for adoption of a brain-death definition that the new clinical indicators of brain death are simply refinements of the traditional cardiovascular indicators for the state of death.

10. A point well argued in Becker, "Human Being." See above, p. 44.

Brain Death as a New Standard

What is lodged in the lower brain is not Capacity S but *neural* capacity for spontaneous respiration and heartbeat. The second argument seeks to provide justification for attaching special importance to this source of machine independence. Two grounds have, in fact, been independently advanced. The first is that brain death is, as a matter of medical fact, soon followed by death of the living system as a whole. The second sees brain death itself as the death of that system.[11] Neither ground is sufficient.

The first is easily dispatched. As Becker observed, "though the loss of one vital function (say loss of the capacity to eliminate wastes) may inevitably *bring about* death, it does not constitute death by itself."[12] Brain death portends bodily death, but does not constitute it. The interval during which a brain-dead patient can be maintained by artificial life-supports is at present quite limited, a fact which Lamb cites in support of a brain-death definition of death; but surely it could be extended, perhaps indefinitely.[13] It is difficult to see why the brevity of the interval should have any bearing on the definition of death. There are a host of medical conditions which, given the current power of medicine, also inevitably lead to death of the system as a whole, just as renal failure did only a few years ago. There was and is no temptation to regard the onset of these conditions as the occasion of death, and, failing further argument, this judgment extends naturally to the brain.[14]

---

11. As Black notes in "Brain Death," these two grounds have given rise to two other kinds of validation studies for brain-death indicators. Those interested in the role of brain death in causing so-called somatic death (death of the rest of the body) have been concerned to demonstrate that somatic death is inevitable once the appropriate indications of brain death appear. Those emphasizing the central place of the brain in the body system are concerned to learn just when the brain disintegrates; what happens to the rest of the body, and when, is treated as immaterial.

12. Becker, "Human Being," p. 42.

13. See Lamb, "Diagnosing Death," p. 174; Black, "Brain Death."

14. There is a series of classic eighteenth-century experiments by LeGallois on rabbit fetuses and pups which makes this point forcibly. LaGallois noted that if these organisms were decapitated above the pneumogastric nerve, the body of the organism remained alive for a period of time equal to that required for suffocation to occur in an organism at that developmental level. For

The other ground for attaching special importance to death of the
(lower) brain, its alleged central role in the functioning body system,
purports to offer a way of distinguishing brain death from other mis-
fortunes which may eventually be fatal. The contention here is that
the brain is more than merely one vital organ among others; in some
important sense it *is* the body system. Lamb states:

> Since the brain stem, not the heart, is recognized as the specific
> area which regulates all vital processes, it follows that after brain
> stem death the heart and other organs can never function again
> naturally. . . . The recognition that the brain stem, not the heart,
> is the central vital agency suggests a recent "paradigm shift" with-
> in the medical profession.[15]

Lamb then proceeds to document the shift to a definition of death
based on brain death—even in patients with hearts still beating—on
the part of several eminent medical specialists.

Lamb's argument deserves careful attention, not least because the
almost universal acceptance of the death of the lower brain as a definition of death in the medical community might seem to invoke the
authority of expert opinion. We shall question this authority.

The argument involves *inter alia* two steps, both of which we find
questionable. First, that a paradigm shift has occurred among scientists; and second, that this gives the rest of us reason to identify death
with brain death.

The problem with the first step lies in what is promised by the term
"paradigm shift." If this is more than mere phrase-mongering, we will
want evidence that there has been some sort of theoretical crisis in
medical science which preceded the alleged shift. We must see medical
science in theoretical crisis, analogous to other critical junctures in

---

very young rabbits, this was a period of several hours! Thus, the proximal cause
of death in each case was asphyxiation, not the decapitation which produced it.
The moral is obvious. If there is nothing peculiar in maintaining that these decapitated bodies, though waning, were still alive, there is nothing peculiar about
maintaining the same position vis-à-vis brain-dead organisms so long as we are
constrained to consider biological considerations alone. For an account of the
LeGallois experiments, see Solomon Diamond, *The Roots of Psychology* (New
York: Basic Books, 1974), pp. 41-44.

15. Lamb, "Diagnosing Death," pp. 146-147.

the history of science, replete with rival comprehensive theories which appear to be incommensurable. But there are none here. As Lamb himself states, the essential scientific facts were all quite well known before anyone gave any thought to changing the definition of death:

> There was, and still is, no doubt concerning the causal relationship between cerebral death and a cessation of the heartbeat. However, it was then (i.e., before the new definition became popular) maintained that death came only with the latter.[16]

Scientists command autonomy in setting some definitions, whether in the course of paradigm shifts or in ordinary science. If, as has happened in the history of science, a chemist wants to change the definition of "acid" to suit theoretical needs, it is up to him and his peers to decide the issue. The revised definition of acid is correct if it augments predictive and explanatory power, and this is a matter in which only the scientist is expert; the rest of us accept the redefinition on faith. The change in the definition of death, however, does not seem to be the sort of response to scientific needs that commands our allegiance. Many of the specialists supporting the change are not scientists at all in the narrow sense of being theory-builders, as they would have to be if we are to be bound to follow their example. They are, rather, medical practitioners. And even those scientists who support this change might not be doing so in their role as theory-builders, since they may simply be responding to the practitioner's statement of need for a definition which facilitates the acquisition of fresh organs and of more room in the intensive care units. To accept Lamb's argument we would need to see new scientific laws formulated or other evidence of the new definition's theoretical, as opposed to moral or practical, utility. Without such evidence, recent wholesale change of opinion within the medical community tells us nothing more than that many physicians have chosen to pronounce brain-dead patients dead.

The reader may feel that even if Lamb's appeal to authority fails to establish the centrality of the brain in the body's system of life-functions, that role is intuitively clear. Certainly the brain's work is

16. Ibid., p. 147.

different from that of any other vital organ. It is the organizer, the integrator; the other organs form the work-force regulated by its commands. And, as Becker points out, the body's life is surely a matter of *systemic* functioning: the continued interaction of a hierarchy of biological and chemical subsystems.[17] What we need is a criterion for determining death of the system; and what better candidate than loss of the command center which maintains systemic integration?

A more careful assessment of the lower brain's role, however, does not support the conclusion that brain death constitutes the cessation of systemic functioning. The fact that the lower brain is the element in the system which keeps other elements acting as a system does not make its continued functioning essential. It is still one among many organs, and, like other organs, could conceivably be replaced by an artificial aid which performed its function. The respirators and other life-supports which maintain body functioning after lower brain death collectively constitute a sort of artificial lower brain, and development of a more perfect mechanical substitute is merely a technological problem. When the lower brain's job is performed by these substitutes, the body's life-system continues to function as a system. The nonessential character of brain death may be brought out by some mechanical analogies: the heating system in a home can continue to function even after its thermostat fails, so long as the furnace is turned on and off manually (or by a substitute machine); an airplane continues to fly even after the autopilot fails if human pilots are able to take control. The source of control is not important; what matters is whether the job is done. The artificial life-supports now in use perform the brain's work rather poorly, as shown by the rapidity with which death of the body usually follows brain death; but not so poorly that the artificially maintained system is no system at all.[18]

17. Becker, "Human Being," p. 42.
18. In denying the relevance of lower brain death in determining death of the body, we follow Becker; we have been concerned here to defend him against Lamb. Were it not for our views on the identity of the brain-dead patient, we would also endorse his positive view that "a human organism is dead when, for whatever reason, the system of those reciprocally dependent processes which assimilate oxygen, metabolize food, eliminate wastes, and keep the organism in relative homeostasis are arrested in a way which the organism itself cannot reverse" ("Human Being," p. 42). Except for the final clause concerning spon-

Thus permanent cessation of lower brain functioning, which is the event known as brain death in the medical literature on the subject, does not mark the moment of death. Indeed, it does not even bear on the question of whether the patient is alive or dead, for any of the reasons found in the medical literature. Just how these arguments miss their mark so badly will be discussed later in this essay.

II. THE MORAL ARGUMENTS

It is morally right to discontinue care of a brain-dead patient. Does this show that brain-dead patients are dead? The answer depends on what one takes the activity of defining death to be. One often cited paper states that

> when we speak of human death . . . we are making a statement with policy implications. We are saying that it is now appropriate to behave towards the individual in a different way. . . . It is appropriate to begin burial ritual and for the deceased's friends and family to begin the mourning process. . . . If the individual is a holder of public office, say, the President of the United States, the Vice President would assume the office of the President. Thus, human death is a social and moral concept quite beyond the biological. . . . The only reason the definition of death receives any attention at all in the realm of public policy is that the term summarizes and legitimates what might be called "death behavior," a radically different set of social relationships and actions.[19]

This passage suggests that to redefine death is to call for new patterns of "death behavior." If declaring a patient dead upon final cessation of breathing amounted to calling for burial and mourning at that time,

---

taneous reversal, the fundamental idea is sound: bodily death consists of functional disintegration. This definition is appropriately vague; it cannot be used to specify an instant of bodily death in most cases, but it serves to rule out a host of illegitimate candidates.

19. Robert M. Veatch, "The Whole-Brain Oriented Concept of Death: An Out-Moded Philosophical Formulation," *Journal of Thanatology* 3 (1975): 13-30. Our continuation of the argument is not meant to represent Veatch's view since our development of this argument is not entirely consonant with his. We endorse Veatch's conclusions and our arguments are complementary to his (though see below, fn. 28). See his *Death, Dying and the Biological Revolution*, chaps. 1-2.

then to pronounce death upon brain death would be to prescribe these practices at the earlier time. Presumably, then, on this view, the way to decide when death occurs is to determine when "death behavior" should begin.

"Death behavior" at the bedside might include mourning, turning off life-support equipment, and removing vital organs for transplantation. Ordinarily there will be little point to delay these acts past the time of brain death, at least not for the patient's sake. Roland Puccetti writes:

> If someone suggested to me that my body might survive death of the neocortex for several months or years, provided it were fed and cleaned properly, etc., that would have no greater appeal to me than preservation of my appendix in a bottle of formaldehyde. For in the sense in which life has value for human beings, I would have been dead all that time.[20]

Taken to mean that life would be no more valuable to the patient than death, there can be no nonreligious objection to this assessment. The brain-dead patient has no capacity for happiness, has no interests, and arguably has no rights. Further attempts to maintain the patient's functional integrity would do him no good and are not morally required of us. The question to be answered, however, is whether the moral proposition that maintenance of the brain dead preserves nothing of value and may be ceased when convenient shows that the brain dead are dead. Many of the medical articles on brain death seem to suggest that it does. There is little real argument of any kind for regarding the brain dead as dead, but the authors regularly mention the pointlessness of maintaining those in irreversible coma and the difficulties for the transplant surgeon caused by waiting for breathing to stop. These concerns clearly motivate the redefinition—again, no new *scientific* data appeared to support the shift—and, in the absence of other argument, seem to appear to the medical authors to justify the redefinition as well.[21] This view of redefinition is explicitly stated by one philosopher:

20. Roland Puccetti, "The Conquest of Death," *The Monist* 59 (1976): 252.
21. If the chief medical impetus for recognizing brain death as death was a moral one, why would the medical criteria for brain death focus on death of

The only way of choosing (between competing definitions of death) is to decide whether or not we attach any value to the preservation of someone irreversibly comatose. Do we value 'life' even if unconscious, or do we value life only as a vehicle for consciousness?[22]

This account of the task of defining death, however, has unacceptable, even absurd, consequences. If our society came to value sports so much that the cripple's sedentary existence was thought to have no value, we would hardly find it congenial to reclassify the lame as dead. In any case, the value of life often drops well before brain death; years before, in some cases of senility. Indeed, many of us would prefer death over continued existence at the level of some profoundly retarded, institutionalized human beings. For all that, there is no temptation to say that these human beings are dead. When they do die, the change is obvious. A reclassification of healthy, profoundly retarded humans as dead would amount to ontological gerrymandering.

Thus the account of defining death which is assumed by the moral arguments is a faulty one, and a source of its error is the way in which the speech act of pronunciation of death is construed. It is certainly true that a person who pronounces a patient dead usually acts differ-

---

the *whole* brain rather than on death of the upper brain alone? The patient whose upper brain is lost has, after all, a life just as low in quality as that of the patient whose whole brain is gone. Medical articles are mostly silent on this issue. An exception is *The Lancet*'s editorial on the occasion of a statement on brain death by the Conference of Royal Colleges and Faculties of the United Kingdom. Their remark that "How long life support should be provided for such survivors of brain damage is a harrowing question, but vegetative patients are not brain dead and the questions of ethics and of the use of resources are different" (13 November 1976, p. 1065) reaffirms the focus on lower rather than higher, brain death, but does not explain the reasons for this focus. The tests for whole brain death were more reliable than those for upper brain death alone, but recent articles disavow this as the reason. Our conversations with medical specialists give us the impression that physicians, so used to attempting to restore the body to functional integrity, cannot bring themselves to pronounce death upon a breathing body which maintains itself with only nutritional and custodial care. Our diagnosis, then, is that moral concern to let the patients lapse, constrained by tradition, caused the physicians to adopt an otherwise unmotivated attitude of respect for the lower brain, identifying its continued functioning with life itself.

22. Jonathan Glover, *Causing Death and Saving Lives* (Middlesex, 1977), p. 45.

ently and expects others to do likewise. But it does not follow that to pronounce a patient dead *is* to state an intention to act differently and to call upon others to follow suit. The conclusion does not follow, even if the sole motives of the person pronouncing death are the statement of intent and the prescription to others. The argument conflates three aspects of speech acts: what is said, the effects of saying it, and the motives for saying it. Two speakers can presumably agree on whether a patient has died even if they endorse different sorts of mourning practices; indeed, even if one of them thinks the practices should begin before death, or only after a decent interval. And, of course, the speaker's intent in pronouncing death may be just to inform his listeners about the condition of the deceased, with no intention of prescribing any practice.

The reason that pronouncing death *seems* to be prescribing termination of care, and the reason that citing the moral advantages of medical abandonment *seems* to be a way of arguing for a redefinition of death as brain death, is that certain moral premises are simply assumed without question or argument: one is that there is no point to giving medical care to the dead and the other is that life should always be preserved. If these positions are abandoned, the pressure to change the definition of death is immediately relieved. We have only to realize that the moment of pulling the plug need not be the moment of death to see that defining death is a different job from deciding when it is best to remove the life-support systems. The heart-lung definition of death did not, and could not, itself, have required pointless maintenance of the brain dead. That severe prescription emerges only when we add the premise that the living must not be abandoned. What the moral arguments show, then, is not that the brain dead are dead but that the brain dead need not be cared for. The moral argument addresses a moral issue which is, unfortunately, confused by many with the task of defining death. Our argument in Section III supports the redefinition, not by demonstrating that the brain dead have a worthless existence, but by showing that they have no existence at all.

III. An Ontological Argument

To state that an ailing patient, Jones, is still alive, is in fact to make two claims; the second of which is usually taken for granted. One is that the patient is alive. The other is that the patient is (remains) *Jones*.[23] It is natural to assume that the living patient, who entered the hospital as Jones, must still be Jones (who else could it be?).[24] But we will show that this is mistaken. If we do establish that the patient, even if alive, is not Jones, and if no one else is Jones, then we will have established that Jones does not exist. And this, of course, establishes that Jones is dead. *Jones*' death thus occurs *either* at the time that the patient dies, if the patient has remained Jones; *or* at the time the patient ceased to be Jones, whichever comes first. If, as we contend, the patient ceased to be Jones at the time of brain death, then Jones' brain death is Jones' death.[25] Thus, if the loss of capacity for mental activity which occurs at brain death constitutes death, it is not for moral reasons, nor for biological reasons, but for *ontological* reasons.[26]

We need, then, to show that the patient ceases to be Jones when brain death strips the body of its psychological traits. We accomplish this by drawing a corollary about brain death from what we believe

23. The term "patient" is used neutrally to designate the entity in the hospital bed. For a discussion of the relation of existence and identity, see Roderick Chisholm, "Coming into Being and Passing Away," in Stuart F. Spicker and H. Tristram Englehardt, eds., *Philosophical Medical Ethics: Its Nature and Significance* (Dordrecht, Holland, 1977), especially p. 171.

24. That brain-dead patients can nevertheless be alive is argued in Section I, above.

25. It is worth emphasizing that we are not speaking of two distinct events, loss of identity and death, which occur in the life of every individual. Once Jones is no longer the living entity we call "the patient," Jones is gone and dead. That his body lives or dies is immaterial. As Becker himself notes ("Human Being," p. 43), the continued life of organs and other entities which were once a part of a living person does not constitute continued life of that person. What matters is whether these tissues *are* that person. Indeed, Jones would be dead, even if his living body were to become another person—assuming, as we shall shew, that such talk makes sense. This shows that the issue is not whether the patient is *a* person after brain death. It is whether the patient is *that* person, Jones.

26. Gareth Matthews offers an ontological argument for brain death in his "Life and Death as the Arrival and Departure of the Psyche," *American Philosophical Quarterly* 16, no. 2 (April 1979): 151-157. Matthews' argument, which proceeds from a neo-Aristotelian notion of *psyche* distinct from current conceptions of "person," identifies death of an organism with the loss of the capacity for self-regulation in the way distinctive of its kind. We find his proposal unsuccessful; a comprehensive examination of Matthews' position would not fall within the scope of this article.

to be the correct theory of personal identity.[27] In what follows, we sketch the theory briefly, emphasizing the role which the theory attributes to the brain function. Then we state the corollary and use it to show that the criteria of personal identity thus derived do not permit identity to survive the kinds of changes which brain death involves. The result justifies a definition of death as brain death.[28]

27. The theory is essentially the view developed by John Perry in a series of articles; see his contributions to his edited volume *Personal Identity* (Berkeley and Los Angeles: University of California Press, 1975) and to Amelie Rorty, ed., *The Identities of Persons* (Berkeley and Los Angeles: University of California Press, 1976); and his review of Bernard Williams' *Problems of the Self* in *Journal of Philosophy* 73, no. 13 (15 July 1976): 416-428. Bernard Gert's "Personal Identity and the Body," *Dialogue*, September 1971, pp. 458-478, from which we also learned much, is in important respects similar. A similar theory is embodied in Jewish law, according to Rabbi Azriel Rosenfeld, who has noted its importance for the brain-death controversy; see his "The Heart, the Head, and the Halakhah," *New York State Journal of Medicine* (15 October 1970): 2615-2619.

28. The notion that the brain-dead patient has "ceased to exist as a person" (see fn. 3, above) has both a moral and an ontological interpretation. The moral claim is simply that the patient's life now lacks the features that make life more valuable for people than death. Our ontological claim is that the person who entered the hospital, he whose body is now brain dead, no longer exists (though his body or some of its parts may both exist and live). Robert Veatch, in his *Death, Dying and the Biological Revolution* holds that "to define the death of a human being, we must recognize the characteristics that are essential to humanness. . . . We use the term *death* to mean the loss of what is essentially significant to an entity—in the case of man, the loss of humanness" (p. 26). "To ask what is essentially significant to a human being is a philosophical question— a question of ethical and other values. Many elements make human beings unique—their opposing thumbs, their possession of rational souls . . . and so on. Any concept of death will depend directly upon how one evaluates these qualities" (pp. 29-30). This seems to be a hybrid: moral considerations dictating our ontological conclusion. Veatch conducts his search for what is "essentially human" and "essential to man's nature" by contrasting various "traditions" ("the empiricalist philosophical tradition seems to be represented in the emphasis on consciousness. . . . At least in the Western tradition, man is seen as an essentially social animal," p. 41), by drawing upon his own and others' intuitions on man's essence, and by citing perceived moral dangers of adopting the views he opposes.

It would be hard to argue for or against this view except by citing one's own intuitions on "man's nature," if any. We avoid the evident difficulties of this approach by constructing a step-by-step argument using the intuitive "data" on personal identity drawn on by Locke and his successors. Though our argument, like Veatch's, appeals in the end to intuitions, it appeals to conceptual intuitions, not moral ones, on which there is considerable consensus, and which are used to test a concept (personal identity) which is considerably better defined

Accounts of Personal Identity

It will seem to some—particularly to philosophers familiar with the literature on personal identity—that there exists a very short argument proving that brain-dead patients are not identical to the persons who once were associated with their bodies. Bernard Gert states:

> . . . if a body does not have any psychological features, then it is not a person, and hence the question of personal identity cannot even arise.[29]

This argument, however, must be recognized as an enthymeme, a full statement of which involves the acknowledgment of two quite substantial metaphysical assumptions. The first of these is an account of what is essential for an individual to belong to a certain kind; in the present case, the claim is that an entity is a person only if it has psychological properties. The second assumption is that it is essential for the continued existence of an individual that it remain a member of the kind to which it belongs. Otherwise, although having the capacity for psychological states might be essential to being a person, it could simply be the case that being a person, like being a musician, was a property that a given individual could acquire or lose in the course of a lifetime without ceasing to be the same individual. Each of these assumptions is notoriously controversial. There is nothing approaching a definitive account of the essence of personhood. And apparent counterexamples to the second assumption abound in nature: a bit of radioactive uranium, for example, may decay and become lead without ceasing to exist.[30] Indeed, on some accounts of what a person is, even persons come into the world as non-persons and, retaining their identity, enter that category upon suitable psychological development. Thus at least one boundary of that kind is permeable.

The approach we take here permits us to remain agnostic on the

---

than Veatch's "human existence." Our individual-essentialism is, relative to Veatch's (and others') kind-essentialism, better methodology if not better metaphysics.

29. Gert, "Personal Identity and the Body," pp. 475-476.

30. Berent Enç, "Natural Kinds and Linnaean Essentialism," *Canadian Journal of Philosophy* 5, no. 1 (1 September 1975): 83-102. See also Marjorie Price, "Identity through Time," *Journal of Philosophy* 74, no. 4 (April 1977): 201-217.

issue of kind-essentialism and on whether membership in a kind is essential to retention of identity. We offer instead an argument which establishes a claim about the essential properties of a given *individual*. The claim is that the continued possession of certain psychological properties by means of a certain causal process is an essential requirement for any given entity to be identical with the individual who is Jones. Thus, we can afford to remain uncommitted on whether persons are essentially beings with psychological properties and on whether Jones is essentially a person. We demonstrate instead that Jones, whatever kind of entity he is, is essentially an entity with psychological properties. Thus, when brain death strips the patient's body of all its psychological traits, Jones ceases to exist.

What is required to show that Jones is an individual who essentially possesses certain psychological capacities is an adequate account of personal identity. The literature on this topic generally assumes that certain individuals are identifiable as persons and then gives an account of the criteria according to which a person existing at one time is to be identified with one existing at a later time. For convenience of exposition, we will continue to talk as though the individuals we pick out are persons, but this will not affect the force of our argument. We need only claim that in normal cases we are able to identify the individual Jones (whether or not he is a person) in order to show that this individual's identity is essentially connected with the possession of certain psychological properties.

Two sorts of personal identity criteria have been proposed. One concerns continuity and connectedness of personality, memory, and other mental phenomena; the other stresses spatio-temporal continuity of the physical body. On the "mentalist" view, two "person-stages" are stages of the same person, just in case the latter is a continuation of the earlier personality and can remember what the earlier one has done.[31] The body-continuity view makes no such requirement; having the same body is sufficient and necessary.

The mentalist's basic argument is the apparent conceivability of

31. A person-stage is a person in a given time interval. A person *simpliciter* is a series of person-stages. The problem of personal identity, thus conceived, is to state the criteria determining which person-stages are stages of the same entity.

body-switching. We can, the mentalist asserts, readily imagine persons coming to inhabit other person's bodies, or switching bodies between them. It certainly seems possible to imagine oneself waking up in another's body. We might have a hard time convincing others who we were, but we feel that we should know it in an instant. The fact that our body might be unfamiliar would be beside the point from the subjective point of view. When we narrate these examples as we usually do, it is plain that we are using a mentalist criterion of personal identity. To the extent that the descriptions of events in these examples are intuitively correct, argues the mentalist, we have established the soundness of the mentalist criterion.

The body-continuity theorists, however, have an effective counter to this argument. What is disputed is not whether these examples can be imagined, but how they ought to be interpreted. Let us suppose that a person *did* wake up feeling that he was Jones, but had a new body, or that two persons seemed able to remember events which had happened in the lives of the persons who had heretofore had the other's body. This does not show that a transfer of bodies has occurred. The subjective phenomenon might be delusive. Many persons have thought they were Napoleon or some other person; they may even have known enough about the other's life and personality to mimic the other person convincingly. If Jones and Smith woke up, each claiming to be the other, this folie à deux would simply be the situation which the mentalist mistakenly calls a body-switch. The difficulty for the mentalist is that an additional criterion of personal identity must be found, one which would establish that the memories are not delusional. But the surest criterion for genuine memory is that the remembered event be one which happened in the rememberer's own history. The circularity is apparent.

Can the mentalist show that the putative identity changes in the body-transfer examples are not merely identity-preserving changes of psychological qualities? Not unless the examples are narrated in greater detail; everything that happens in the example mentioned above is consistent with a body-theorist's interpretation. But the mentalist can elaborate the story in a way that rules out this possibility and thus demonstrates the conceptual possibility of a person being serially identical with distinct bodies.

This consists of making clear *why* the narrated changes occur. The body theorist's counter-construal is silent on this point, but one's imagination can supply a range of possible causes. Jones might have been subjected to brainwashing by someone who wanted him to feel and act like Smith. Or Jones might have endured a psychotic episode in which the character of his friend, Smith, provided the organizing motif for his delusions. Or the delusions might coincidentally have formed a coherent personality and imagined life-history which duplicated that of Smith, a total stranger.

Other explanations could be dreamed up, but we need not extend this list. What is important for our purposes is the fact that the body-theorist's counter-construal appears plausible *only because* the alleged body-transfer narrative permits us to assume the applicability of one or another of these explanations. But suppose a body-switch narrative could be told in sufficient detail to preclude the typical body-theorist interpretations. If all these possible explanations of the qualitative changes were ruled out, we would have no reason to suppose that mere qualitative change had occurred. Then, unless the body-theorist is prepared to offer, in addition to a reconstrual of identity change as qualitative change, some new and powerful *explanation* for the latter, his argument will fail to convince. We would look for some other account.

The likely alternative, of course, would be that of the mentalist: these changes occurred because the persons switched bodies. This account, too, can be convincing only upon the assumption that an adequate explanation of events is offered, that is, an explanation of how (what we want to call) Jones' assumption of Smith's body occurred. And the explanation or explanations which would be acceptable here will characteristically be different from those which would have been accepted as accounting for personality changes. In fact, the explanations can be enumerated. If one believes in a Cartesian soul, the body-transfer must involve some sort of incorporeal unhitching from Jones' body and subsequent rehitching onto Smith's. The mentalist, however, is not tied to Cartesian dualism. Even if he grants that all mental events are physical events, there is a way that an event in Smith's life could come to be remembered by a person with Jones' body. Since memory is (presumably) stored in the brain, and since recall is (presumably) an activity of the brain, the switching of bodies

between Smith and Jones could be brought about by transplanting
Smith's brain into Jones' body and vice versa.[32]

To put the point in general terms: body-transfer will have occurred
if and only if the sort of explanation of the continuity of a person's
psychological properties is the same as that which explains this continuity in ordinary life histories (that is, those involving no body
transfer). Personal identity presupposes a characteristic causal tie
between person-stages (what the cause is, exactly, depends on what,
empirically, causes psychological continuity). Indeed, this causal tie
is the criterion of personal identity.[33]

Persons can switch bodies, then, if the causal connections between
the psychological events in the respective bodies are the same as those
which normally obtain among the psychological events which occur in
the history of a normal human body. We know these causes to operate
primarily within the neural system; specifically the brain. Thus it is
that brain-transplantation would also constitute transfer of a person
from one body to another. *Personal* identity, then, seems to be con-
gruent with *brain* identity. This proves to be a happy result in con-

32. That a materialist view of mind and person can coexist with our view
that persons cease to exist before their bodies do is denied by Saul Kripke
("Naming and Necessity," in G. Harman and D. Davidson, eds., *Semantics of
Natural Languages*, Dordrecht, 1972, p. 334 and fn. 73). Kripke, after attacking
a crude materialist view, admits that a sophisticated materialist cum mentalist
would identify the person with a body *whose brain enjoyed the proper physical
organization.* Kripke claims that even this latter approach falls prey to modal
difficulties, but he does not attempt to show this, and we have not been persuaded of any incompatability of materialism with our position by the objections he does offer (for a fuller treatment of Kripke's views; see Fred Feldman,
"Kripke on the Identity Theory," *Journal of Philosophy* 71, no. 24 (October
1974): 666 ff. The outcome of this debate is not relevant to our present purposes, however. Although we have spoken of memory as though it is a brain
process, thus suggesting support of a mind-brain identity thesis, all we require
is that mental life be nomologically dependent on brain-functioning and that
the capacity for consciousness should follow the undamaged brain wherever it
might go. This we take modern neuroscience to have established beyond controversy.

33. Body-continuity theorists aim their fire at examples which, like Locke's,
leave the causes unspecified. The brain-transplantation variants escape their
attention (a point made by Perry in his review of B. Williams, *Problems of the
Self*, and by Gert, "Personal Identity and the Body") and the various arguments
used against the Lockean cases score no points against them.

sideration of several of the familiar cases. Consider, for example, a decapitated person whose head and body are each sustained by high-technology medicine.[34] If the head can communicate with us, and shows psychological connectedness and continuity with the erstwhile person, there can be little doubt that it *is* that person and the body is not.

But the equation of personal and brain identity needs to be qualified. Suppose that during a brain-transplantation experiment, the brain is inadvertently subjected to a process which removes all memory traces from it; indeed, "unwires" the brain so completely that the owner's entire complement of mental traits and capacities is permanently erased.[35] We feel no urge to regard the individual resulting from placing the unwired brain in a "new" body as the person previously associated with the brain. Brain identity alone is insufficient for personal identity. The reason for this follows immediately from the account given above: the ordinary causal processes which link events in a personal history involve more than spatio-temporal

34. Or, substitute brain for head, assuming that the brain can be hooked up to sensory devices and provided with some means of self-expression. An early treatise on medical jurisprudence, *Manual of Medical Jurisprudence and State Medicine* by M. Ray (London, 1836, 2d ed.), p. 499, stated that "individuals who are apparently destroyed in a sudden manner, by certain wounds, diseases or even decapitation, are not really dead, but are only in conditions incompatible with the persistence of life." On our own view, the body may well be *alive*—so may the head—but only one is the person who was once whole.

Becker, "Human Being," p. 47, says: "Bizarre questions may be raised, of course. Is a human brain separated from its body and kept 'functioning' a human being? . . . I admit to being at a loss for a reply to such cases, let alone an answer." Again, Becker has addressed the wrong question: we want to know not (only) if the brain is *a* human being, but *which* human being, where the "human being" means "person." Becker would presumably find our question unanswerable as well; we simply regard the case as more easily conceivable than Becker professes to do. On the conceivability of isolated brains having psychological states, see Bernard Gert, "Can a Brain have a Pain," *Philosophy and Phenomenological Research* 27, no. 3 (March 1967): 432-436, and references cited therein. For a case in which such a state may already have existed in an isolated brain, see fn. 19 in Pucetti, "The Conquest of Death."

35. This sort of imagery is, of course, fatuous. We can foresee no reason why a variant which is truer to the facts should not provide the same conclusion, however. Perry refers to this process as a "brain zap" in his review of B. Williams, *Problems of the Self.*

continuity of brain tissue. They also require continuity of certain brain *processes*, carried out through microstructural and microfunctional registrations in the brain tissue. Two body-stages which fail to be linked by continuity of these processes will fail to be stages of the same person, even if identity of the brain is preserved.[36]

Identity and Brain Death

Our argument that personal identity does not survive brain death requires but one further observation. We have throughout this discussion spoken of body transfers, cases in which a person's identity "leaves" one body and "arrives" at another. We have undertaken to state the conditions under which the entire transfer occurs. We have a fortiori stated the conditions under which each component of the transfer occurs; in particular, under which the ceasing to be associated with one body occurs. When a brain and its ongoing ordinary physiological processes are removed from one body to another, personal identity follows. But it is not necessary that the functioning brain reach its destination for identity to have vacated the donor body. If the brain fails to find a new home and is destroyed, the person's history comes to an end; the continued life functioning of the person's former body is as irrelevant to the issue as it would be had the brain been lodged in the intended new body and the resulting person continued to live.

We submit that, in quite ordinary clinical circumstances, a brain-dead body has similarly been stripped of the identity of the formerly associated person; and this holds true even if that body continues to live. It is not necessary that the brain actually be removed for personal identity to quit the body. The reason that brain removal cancels personal identity in the donor body, after all, is that the resulting

36. Contrast this case from Gert's "Personal Identity and the Body": Jones is hypnotized and made to think, feel, and otherwise resemble Smith in all mental respects. Then the brain is transplanted into Smith's body. The resulting individual is Jones, even though it is psychologically similar to Smith and has Smith's body. The reason is that, in this case, the causal relations between body-stages (hypnosis as well as transplantation) are personal-identity preserving. (In fact, this case involves considerable philosophical license: if hypnosis or other psychological procedures could produce the vast changes alleged here, our concept of personal identity would be considerably different from what it is.)

body cannot thereafter have the kind of causal relation to earlier person-body stages which is required for the personal identity to hold. Brain death has the same result. Indeed, it is unimaginable that the identity question could be much affected by the physical removal of a permanently malfunctioning (and possibly liquified) brain from a living brain-dead body. Brain death and brain removal have much the same result; the dead brain serves only to add bulk to the body if left intact. If, as has been established above, removal of the conscious, functioning brain leaves us with a body not identical to the person formerly associated with it, surely removal of a dead brain leaves just the same thing; and no more remains when the brain dies in place.

Personal identity can, in theory, survive an operation in which the brain is removed from the body; it will lodge either in the brain (if suitably maintained) or in a new host body. If the brain dies, whether in its customary body or elsewhere, so does the person whose brain it is. The continuation of life in the body is immaterial in deciding this question.[37] That body is no more Jones than would be the continuation of the life of each of his cells in Petri dishes, or of each of his organs in the proper solution, after an ordinary death; it is merely better integrated tissue and organ functioning. We have, then, an argument for regarding a person's brain death as that person's death tout court which avoids both covert moral prescriptions and spurious appeals to the authority of biomedical science. The death of persons, unlike that of bodies, regularly consists in their ceasing to exist.

We have now only to relate our ontological argument to the brain-death controversy. We have argued, following other personal identity theorists, that a given person ceases to exist with the destruction of whatever processes there are which normally underlie that person's psychological continuity and connectedness. We know these processes are essentially neurological, so that irreversible cessation of upper-brain functioning constitutes the death of that person. Whole-brain death is also death for persons, but only because whole-brain death is partly comprised of upper-brain death. Tests for either will be tests for death.

37. The same would be true if a new person's brain, carrying that person's brain structure and processes, were transplanted into the body. The result would be a living person, but not the person, now dead, whose body it formerly was.

Of course, our view does not imply that a person dies with his last moment of consciousness. What matters is the preservation of the substrate, not the psychological states which it produces. Hence a person who suffers brain death during sleep dies at the time of brain death, not the time of onset of sleep. Similarly, a person in a persistent coma might be alive if enough of the brain remained structurally and functionally intact.

Further, it does not follow from our argument that all humans lacking the substrate of consciousness are dead. Anencephalic infants are lacking at birth the cortical material necessary for the development of cognitive functioning and, arguably, consciousness. Still, due to possession of a functioning brain stem, they may have spontaneous breathing and heartbeat, and a good suck. Accounts which simply identified life with upper brain function would have to classify these infants as dead, which they obviously are not. We, on the other hand, need only point out that the identity criteria for the anencephalic, never-to-be conscious infant do not involve causal substrates for higher level psychological continuity. The conditions for life and existence will be those of human bodies rather than those of persons.

Finally, we emphasize that our argument, requiring no moral premises, is not sufficient to yield moral conclusions. We show that the brain dead are dead, but it does not follow that brain death is the appropriate moment to turn off ventilators or to remove organs. These acts, and other "death behavior" might be in order at some earlier time, as circumstances dictate. The relationship between defining and pronouncing death, and discontinuing care will receive further discussion in our section on the legal definition of death.

IV. The Legal Definition of Death

We have argued for the definition of death as brain death, and hence have no major quarrel with the current trend toward that definition in statutory and case law.[38] But neither, in our opinion, should those who

38. Two unresolved problems of detail pose problems for those writing brain-death statutes. One is how to specify medical criteria of brain death in a way that assures a minimum of false positives. The second is the harmonious accommodation of the quite different criteria which will be used by physicians and coroners called upon to pronounce death in settings as diverse as intensive

reject our arguments and who cleave to the traditional heart-lung
definition. The reasons we will give for this are moral ones. Our
position calls for some explaining, especially in view of our insistence
(in Section II) that moral considerations should be resolutely ignored
in formulating a definition of death.

To Becker, allowing moral considerations to determine a definition
of death is a cowardly evasion:

> Rigging the definition of death . . . while tempting, is an avoidance
> of the real issue. The real issue is whether, and if so when, it is
> moral to give up trying to prolong the patient's life . . . It seems
> best to face this problem directly—by defining when it is permissible
> to give up life-saving efforts—and not to evade the problem by intro-
> ducing an ad hoc definition of death.[39]

But Becker offers no argument to support this last claim. Perhaps he
felt he could assume agreement on the importance of being true to the
facts. If so, his confidence is misplaced. However imperative truth is
in theoretical work, the cardinal virtues of our social institutions are
justice and utility. These will, we feel, attach to a policy that *does*
evade the problem (assuming, for the sake of argument, that it is a
problem) worrying Becker.

Becker feels, as do we, that discontinuation of medical care of
brain-dead patients is morally acceptable, even mandatory. By Becker's
definition of death, such action amounts to giving up life-saving
efforts. If this sort of medical action were to be endorsed by statute
or other governmental sanction, it might take the form of releasing
physicians from the legal obligation to preserve the life of the irreversibly comatose.[40] The standard argument against this sort of policy
is that it threatens a slide down a slippery slope: today we endorse
the withdrawal of care from the comatose; perhaps tomorrow from the
senile, the moderately retarded, the nonproductive. The likelihood of
such a slide is probably impossible to measure with any confidence,

---

care units, accident sites, and cornfields. Neither of these has significant theoretical interest.

39. Becker, "Human Being," pp. 45-46.

40. Since doctors are rarely, if ever, prosecuted for decisions to cease medical
support of the permanently comatose, such a statute might not be needed.

but it surely is not negligible. Some persons now being retained in institutions for the mentally retarded, after all, have a cognitive life not much different from Karen Quinlan's. And the historical precedent (admittedly under vastly different sociopolitical conditions) has already been set.[41]

Whatever danger exists of a drift toward unjustified euthanasia would be significantly lessened if the statute licensing termination of care of brain-dead patients were one which classified them as dead rather than alive; one which, given a heart-lung definition of death, evaded the euthanasia issue. For the public, whether justifiably or not, seems willing to regard brain-dead patients as dead. A brain-death statute thus has the virtue of leaving official public policy on euthanasia, presently quite restrictive, apparently unchanged. This legal step would portend a threat to the senile and retarded only if the public came to think of them as *dead*, an eventuality which is most unlikely. The danger of the slippery slope is, then, blocked by setting a precedent which would be nearly invulnerable to distortion. Since almost all parties to the euthanasia dispute agree that the best (minimum) policy would be one which authorized withdrawal of care of the permanently comatose but no one else, licensing "letting die" by brain-death statute would be an ideal step.

Are there any serious moral objections to such an evasion? The fact that the policy would (in the view of those endorsing the heart-lung definition of death) embody a falsehood may count against it. But public policy should be granted some autonomy in these matters. The question of whether (to take an historical example) tomatoes should be classified as a vegetable or a fruit for tax purposes ought to be decided by political and economic considerations, not by biological ones.[42] It is true that an evasion in brain-death legislation would serve to dampen rather than stimulate public debate on these matters. But given the dangers alleged to be inherent in such debate, this may count against an "honest" statute.[43]

41. Leo Alexander, "Medical Science Under Dictatorship," *New England Journal of Medicine* 241, no. 2 (14 July 1949): 39-47.

42. Though once the rules are set, those adversely affected may try to use a biological argument to reverse the ruling and to advance their interests. See Charles M. Rick, "The Tomato," *Scientific American* 239 (2 August 1978): 76-86.

43. There are two positions which are immune to our argument on public

Those who (mistakenly, in our view) do not agree that brain death *is* death, then, may still have reason to support brain-death legislation authorizing withdrawal of life supports from brain-dead patients. Such support will be automatically coming from those convinced, as we are, that brain dead patients are dead (though, as we argue here, such a conclusion is not always sufficient to dictate public policy). The philosophical arguments determine the truth of the definition but not the morality of propounding it.

V. Death as Brain Death

We have argued that the death of a person's brain is that person's death. Since we believe that the argument we provide constitutes the only grounds for accepting the theoretical definition of death as brain death, it is important to reemphasize the differences between our argument and those which have been most widely accepted.

We have distinguished a number of *biological* arguments for defining death as brain death. They can all be faulted for their focus on the brain stem since (by our argument) it is loss of upper brain function which marks the person's death. Death of the brain stem is no more constitutive of death *simpliciter* than death of the kidneys or of other vital organs. The arguments we have criticized in Section I rest either on unwarranted identification of the brain stem with the

---

policy. We shall state these without any discussion, though both raise important issues deserving greater consideration. First, those who both disagree with our conclusions and believe that it would be a good thing to have a debate leading to a policy of limited euthanasia would not want to take the muted course we advocate. Second, there are those who will be concerned about an important difference between the "tomato" case and the topic of this paper. The justification for the evasive public policy in the present case rests on the assumption that those making policy have made a correct *moral judgment* on a very important topic and that this decision justifies the evasive legislation. There is no comparable moral decision in the tomato case, just prudential considerations, so that no "evasion" arises, merely pragmatic redefinition. Thus, the tactic advocated here, even if it is supported in this case by a correct moral judgment, is implicitly authorizing lawmakers to employ evasive or conceptually mistaken legislation when, in their best judgment, moral considerations lead them to conclude it would be justified. The path advised here may be an instance of a kind of policy making which, even if justified in this individual case taken in isolation, should probably not be encouraged.

body's biosystem as a whole or on erroneous appeals to the authority of medico-legal tradition or current medical opinion. On our view, the central question about death—which state of a person's body constitutes death—is answered in large part by means of a *metaphysical* argument. The only purely "biological" question is how this state can be clinically identified, and it is on this issue—not the former—that we must defer to medical expertise.

The *moral* argument proceeds from the intuition that the existence of the brain-dead patient is without any value to itself or others. Those using this argument construe the definition of death as a prescription of certain actions. The argument is successful in supporting the conclusion that care should be withdrawn from the brain dead. It can even be used to support a statute calling these patients dead. But it in no way shows that the brain dead *are* dead; this issue is never engaged.

Our argument, by contrast, is free of moral premises. The notion of "person" enters in, not because of any moral view concerning what sorts of entities have rights, but because the most likely account of personal identity serves to show that after brain death the person who entered the hospital has literally ceased to exist. Our claim that the person has died, of course, follows immediately from this. The account of personal identity uses as "data" determinations of the identities of persons and bodies in certain circumstances, but involves no testing of moral intuitions. And the moral issues concerning the patient's care are left open.

There is one more point our argument clarifies. It comes as no surprise that the continued capacity for a mental life is what makes our life valuable. Without it, life would not be worth living. But the connection between our having a capacity for a mental life and that life being of value to us is even tighter than many have supposed. For the position we hold here is not simply that a mindless future life would be of no value to us, but that such a life, whatever else might be true of it, could not be ours.

Finally, we have shown that whatever one's stance on the theoretical issues mentioned above, there may be sound moral reasons to support the current trend in public policy which extends the definition of death to include the brain dead. For those who think that brain-dead patients are still alive, this is a moral evasion. But if we wish to keep our official

Brain Death and
Personal Identity

policy on euthanasia strict to avoid any slippery-slope difficulties, it is an ideal evasion. It is extremely implausible that the public, which believes that the brain dead are dead, could ever come to believe that the profoundly retarded or the grossly senile are dead; even though the mental life of some of these may not be much greater than that of brain-dead patients. This would prevent an extension and abuse of the statute which might follow upon (what those not persuaded by our previous arguments would consider) a more straightforward account assessing the "quality of life," one which would involve prescriptions of the form "killing (or 'letting die') is impermissible except when . . . ." And we have noted that public policy is entitled to such autonomy. Brain dead patients are in fact dead but that is not the reason to have their bodies die.

We have tried, then, to deal with the delicate topics of brain death, death, and personal identity, keeping in mind that the spheres of morality, ontology, science, and public policy, while related, are quite distinct. Our solution to the problem, we believe, gives each sphere its due without arrogating the domain of the others.

Daniel Wikler gratefully acknowledges suggestions from those who commented on an ancestor of this essay read at the University of Wisconsin, Georgetown University, and Oberlin College, and from Norman Fost, David Mayo, and Elliott Sober, and thanks the Joseph P. Kennedy, Jr. Foundation for financial support. The present work is a descendant of a union of that paper and a paper by Michael B. Green, who expresses his appreciation for the support of the Minnesota Center for Philosophy of Science and of its Director, Grover Maxwell. Dr. Green also thanks William Winslade, Co-Director of the UCLA Program in Medicine, Law & Human Values, for providing the opportunity to investigate the topic of this essay.

PART II
Health and
Social Policy

NORMAN DANIELS　　　Health-Care Needs
and Distributive Justice

I. Why a Theory of Health-Care Needs?

A theory of health-care needs should serve two central purposes. First, it should illuminate the sense in which we—at least many of us—think health care is "special," that it should be treated differently from other social goods. Specifically, even in societies in which people tolerate (and glorify) significant and pervasive inequalities in the distribution of most social goods, many feel there are special reasons of justice for distributing health care more equally. Some societies even have institutions for doing so. To be sure, others argue it is perverse to single out health care in this way, or that if we have reasons for doing so, they are rooted in charity, not justice. But in any case, a theory of health-care needs should show their connection to other central notions in an acceptable theory of justice. It should help us see what kind of social good health-care is by properly relating it to social goods whose importance is similar and for which we may have a clearer grasp of appropriate distributive principles.

Second, such a theory should provide a basis for distinguishing the more from the less important among the many kinds of things health care does for us. It should tell us which health-care services are "more special" than others. Thus, a broad category of health-services functions to improve quality of life, not to extend or save it. Some of these services restore or compensate for diminished capacities and functions; others improve life quality in other ways. We do draw distinctions about the urgency and importance of such services. Our theory of health-care needs should provide a basis for a reasonable set of such distinctions. If we can assume some scarcity of health-care resources,[1]

---

1. The objection that health-care resources are scarce only because we waste

and if we cannot (or should not) rely just on market mechanisms to al-
locate these resources, then we need such a theory to guide macro-
allocation decisions about priorities among health-care needs.

In short, a theory of health-care needs must come to grips with two
widely held judgments: that there is something especially important
about health care, and that some kinds of health care are more important than others. The philosophical task is to assess, explain, and
justify or modify these distinctions we make about the importance
of different wants, interests, or needs. After considering a preliminary
objection to the claim that we need a theory of health care needs
(Section II), I shall offer an account of basic needs in general (Section III) and health care needs in particular (Section IV). These needs
are important to maintaining normal species functioning, and in turn,
such normal functioning is an important determinant of the range of
opportunity open to an individual. This connection to opportunity
helps clarify the kind of social good health-care is and provides the
basis for subsuming health-care institutions under principles of
distributive justice (Sections V and VI).

II. A PRELIMINARY OBJECTION

Before turning to the theory, I would like to address one objection
to the project as a whole, for there is reason to think that talk about
health-care needs and their priorities both is avoidable and undesirable. The objection, which challenges the assumption that we cannot
rely on medical markets even where there is adequate income redistribution, can be put as follows: Suppose we could agree on a theory of
distributive justice that gives us a notion of a *fair income share*. Then
individuals could protect themselves against the risk of needing health
care by voluntary insurance schemes. Each person would be responsible for buying insurance at a level of protection he or she desires.
No one (except children and the congenitally handicapped) has a
claim on social resources to meet health care needs unless he is prudent enough to buy the relevant insurance (which does not preclude
charity). Resource allocation to meet demand, expressed through

---

money on frivolous things presupposes distinctions which a theory of needs
should illuminate.

varying insurance packages, can be accommodated by the medical market, provided appropriate competitive conditions obtain. In this way there is protection against expensive but rare needs for health care, for which relatively inexpensive insurance can be bought; so too, common but inexpensive services can either be risk-shared through insurance or paid out of pocket without great sacrifice, if preferred. But expensive and potentially common "needs"—for example, to be provided with artificial hearts or to be cryogenically preserved—would not become a drain on social resources since individuals who want protection against the risks of facing them would have to buy expensive insurance out of their own fair shares. This way of meeting health needs does not create a bottomless pit into which we are forced to drain all available social resources.[2]

Sometimes needs-based theories are criticized because they give us too small a claim on social resources, providing only a floor on deprivation.[3] In contrast, the objection we face here warns against granting precedence to the satisfaction of needs because we then allow too great a claim on social resources. I postpone until Section VI considering how a need-based theory can avoid this problem. Similarly, I shall not here defend the assumption that medical markets fail to be acceptable allocative mechanisms.[4] Instead, I would like to suggest that the insurance scheme fails to obviate the need for a theory of health-care needs.

2. I paraphrase Charles Fried, *Right and Wrong* (Cambridge: Harvard, 1978), pp. 126ff. See my comments on Fried's proposal in "Rights to Health Care: Programmatic Worries," *Journal of Medicine and Philosophy* 4, no. 2 (June 1979): 174-191. I ignore here an issue of paternalism which Fried may have wanted to pursue but which is better raised when fair shares are clearly large enough to purchase a reasonable insurance package. Should the premium purchase be compulsory?

3. Needs-based theories cut two ways. Egalitarians use them to criticize the failure of inegalitarian systems to meet basic human needs. Inegalitarians use them to justify providing only minimally for basic needs while allowing significant inequalities above the floor. Here I resist the temptation to respond to the inegalitarian by expanding the category of needs to consume such inequalities.

4. Arrow's classic paper traces the anomalies of the medical market to the uncertainties in it. My analysis has a bearing on the further moral issue, whether health care ought to be marketed even in an ideal market. Cf. Kenneth Arrow, "Uncertainty and the Welfare Economics of Medical Care," *American Economic Review* 53 (1963): 941-973.

The key assumption underlying this scheme is that the prudent citizen will be able to buy a *reasonable* health-care insurance package from his fair share. Such a package can meet the health-care needs it is *reasonable for people to want to be protected against*. However, if some fair shares turn out to be inadequate to pay the premium for such a package, then there is something unacceptable about them. Intuitively, they are not fair to those people. But we can describe such a benefit package, and thus determine minimum constraints on a fair share, only if we already use a notion of basic or reasonable health-care needs, the ones it is rational for a prudent person to insure against. So the "fair share plus insurance" approach only *appears* to avoid talk about health-care needs. Either it must smuggle such a theory in when it arrives at constraints on fair shares, or else it is open to the objection the shares are not fair.

There is another way in which a theory of health-care needs is implicit in the insurance-scheme market approach: the approach puts health-care needs on a par with other wants and preferences and allows them to compete for resources with no constraints other than market mechanisms operating.[5] But such a stance, far from avoiding the need to develop a theory of needs, already *is* a view of health care needs. It sees them as one kind of preference among many, with no special claim on social resources except that which derives from strength of preference. To be sure, where strength of preference is high, needs may be met, but strength may vary in ways that fail to reflect the importance we ought (and usually do) ascribe to health care. Such a market view needs justification, and it is not a justification simply to point to the *existence* of such a market.

III. NEEDS AND PREFERENCES

Not All Preferences are Created Equal

Before turning to health-care needs in particular, it is worth noting that the concept of needs has been in philosophical disrepute, and with

5. The presence of people with preferences for more-than-reasonable coverage may result in inflationary pressures on the premium for "reasonable" insurance packages. So interference in the market is likely to be necessary to protect the adequacy of fair shares.

some good reason. The concept seems both too weak and too strong to get us very far toward a theory of distributive justice. Too many things become needs, and too few. And finding a middle ground seems to involve many of the issues of distributive justice one might hope to resolve by appeal to a clear notion of needs.

It is easy to see why too many things appear to be needs. Without abuse of language, we refer to the means necessary to reach any of our goals as needs. To reawaken memories of Miller's, the neighborhood delicatessen of my childhood, I need only the smell of sour pickles in a barrel. To paint my son's swing set, I need a clean brush.[6] The problem of the importance of needs seems to reduce to the problem of the importance or urgency of preferences or wants in general (leaving aside the fact that not all the things we need are expressed as preferences).

But just as not all preferences are on a par—some are more important than others—so too not all the things we say we need are. It is possible to pick out various things we say we need, including needs for health care, which play a special role in a variety of moral contexts. Taking a cue from T. M. Scanlon's discussion in "Preference and Urgency," we should distinguish *subjective* and *objective* criteria of well-being.[7] We need *some* such criterion to assess the importance of competing claims on resources in a variety of moral contexts. A *subjective* criterion uses the relevant individual's own assessment of how well-off he is with and without the claimed benefit to determine the importance of his preference or claim. An *objective* criterion invokes a measure of importance independent of the individual's own assessment, for example, independent of the *strength* of his preference.

In contexts of distributive justice and other moral contexts, we do *in fact* appeal to some *objective* criteria of well-being. We refuse to

6. For emphasis, we often refer to things we simply desire or want as things we need. Sometimes we invoke a distinction between noun and verb uses of "need," so that not everything we say we need counts as *a need*. Any distinction we might draw between noun and verb uses depends on our purposes and the context and would still have to be explained by the kind of analysis I undertake above.

7. T. M. Scanlon, "Preference and Urgency," *Journal of Philosophy* 77, no. 19 (November 1975): 655-669.

rely solely on subjective ones. If I appeal to my friend's duty of benef-
icence in requesting $100, I will most likely get a quite different reac-
tion if I tell him I need the money to get a root-canal than if I tell him
I need the money to go to the Brooklyn neighborhood of my childhood
to smell pickles in a barrel. Indeed, it is not likely to matter in his
assessment of *obligations* that I strongly *prefer* to go to Brooklyn. Nor
is it likely to matter if I insist I feel a great *need* to reawaken memories
of my childhood—I am overcome by nostalgia. (He might give me the
money for either purpose, but if he gives it so I can smell pickles, we
would probably say he is not doing it out of any duty at all, that he
feels no obligation.) Similarly, if my appeal was directed to some
(even utopian) social welfare agency rather than my friend, it would
adopt objective criteria in assessing the importance of the request
independent of my own strength of preference.

The issue as Scanlon has drawn it, between subjective and objective
standards of well-being, is not just a claim about the *epistemic* status
of our criteria of well-being. He is surely right that we do not rely on
subjective standards of well-being: we do not just accept an individual's assessment of his well-being as the *relevant* measure of his well-
being in important moral contexts. But the issue here is not just that
such a measure is *subjective* and we use an *objective* measure. Nor
is the issue that we may be skeptical about the feasibility of developing an objective interpersonal measure of satisfaction, and so we
use another measure. Suppose we had an intersubjectively acceptable
way of determining individual levels of well-being, where well-being
is viewed as the level of satisfaction of the individual's *full range of
preferences*. That is, suppose we had some deep social-utility function
that enabled us to compare different persons' levels of satisfaction,
given the full-range of their preferences and the social goods they have
available. Such a scale would be the wrong scale to use in a broad
range of moral contexts involving justice and the design of social
institutions—at least it is not just an improvement on the scale we do
in fact use. We would continue to use a far narrower scale of well-
being, one that *does not include the full range of kinds of preferences*
people have. So the real issue behind Scanlon's insightful discussion is the choice between objective *truncated* or selective scales of

well-being and either objective or subjective *full-range* or "satisfaction" scales of well-being.[8] I shall return shortly to consider why the truncated scale *ought to be* (and not just *is*) the measure used in issues of social justice.

One indication that we appeal to an objective, truncated standard is that I might say the root-canal, but not the smell of pickles in a barrel, is something I *really* need (assuming the dentist is right). It is a *need* and not just a desire. The implication is that some of the things we claim to need fall into special categories which give them a weightier moral claim in contexts involving the distribution of resources (depending, of course, on how well-off we already are within those categories of need).[9] Our task is to characterize the relevant categories of needs in a way that *explains* two central properties these special needs have. First, these needs are *objectively ascribable*: we can ascribe them to a person even if he does not realize he has them and even if he denies he has them because his preferences run contrary to the ascribed needs. Second, and of greater interest to us, these needs are *objectively important*: we attach a special weight to claims based on them in a variety of moral contexts, and we do so independently of the weight attached to these and competing claims by the relevant individuals. So our philosophical task is to characterize the class of things we need which has these properties and to do so in such a way that we explain why such importance is attached to them.

Needs and Species-Typical Functioning

One plausible suggestion for distinguishing the relevant needs from all the things we can come to need is David Braybrooke's distinction between "course-of-life needs" and "adventitious needs." *Course-of-life needs* are those needs which people "have all through their lives

8. The difference might not be in the *extent* but in the *content* of the scale. An objective full-range satisfaction scale might be constructed so that some categories of (key) preferences are lexically primary to others; preferences not included on a truncated scale never enter the full-range scale except to break ties among those equally well-off on key preferences. Such a scale may avoid my worries, but it needs a rationale for its ranking. The objection raised here to full-range satisfaction measures applies, I believe, with equal force to happiness or enjoyment measures of the sort Richard Brandt defends in *A Theory of the Good and the Right* (Oxford: Oxford University Press, 1979), chap. 14.

9. See Scanlon, "Preference and Urgency," p. 660.

or at certain stages of life through which all must pass." *Adventitious needs* are the things we need because of the particular contingent projects (which may be long-term ones) on which we embark. Human course-of-life needs would include food, shelter, clothing, exercise, rest, companionship, a mate (in one's prime), and so on. Such needs are not themselves deficiencies, for example, when they are anticipated. But a deficiency with respect to them "endangers the normal functioning of the subject of need *considered as a member of a natural species.*"[10] A related suggestion can be found in McCloskey's discussion of the human and personal needs we appeal to in political argument. He argues that needs "relate to what it would be detrimental to us to lack, *where the detrimental is explained by reference to our natures as men and specific persons.*"[11]

The suggestion here is that the needs which interest us are those things we need in order to achieve or maintain species-typical normal functioning. Do such needs have the two properties noted earlier? Clearly they are objectively ascribable, assuming we can come up with the appropriate notion of species-typical functioning. (So, incidentally, are adventitious needs, assuming we can determine the relevant goals by reference to which the adventitious needs become determinate.) Are these needs objectively important in the appropriate

10. David Braybrooke, "Let Needs Diminish That Preferences May Prosper," in *Studies in Moral Philosophy*, American Philosophical Quarterly Monograph Series, No. 1 (Blackwells: Oxford, 1968), p. 90 (my emphasis). Personal medical services do not count as course-of-life needs on the criterion that we need them all through our lives or at certain (developmental) stages, but they do count as course-of-life needs in that deficiency with respect to them may endanger normal functioning.

11. McCloskey, unlike Braybrooke, is committed to distinguishing a narrower noun use of "need" from the verb use. See J. H. McCloskey, "Human Needs, Rights, and Political Values," *American Philosophical Quarterly* 13, no. 1 (January 1976): 2f (my emphasis). McCloskey's proposal is less clear to me than Braybrooke's: presumably our natures include species-typical functioning but something more as well. Moreover, McCloskey is more insistent than Braybrooke in leaving room for *individual natures*, though Braybrooke at least leaves room for something like this when he refers to the needs that we may have by virtue of individual temperament. The hard problem that faces McCloskey is distinguishing between things we need *to develop our individual natures* and things we come to need in the process of what he calls "self-making," the carrying out of projects one chooses, perhaps in acordance with one's nature but not just by way of developing it.

way? In a broad range of contexts we do treat them as such—a claim I shall not trouble to argue. What is of interest is to see *why* being in such a need category gives them their special importance.

A tempting first answer might be this: whatever our specific chosen goals or tasks, our ability to achieve them (and consequently our happiness) will be diminished if we fall short of normal species functioning. So, whatever our specific goals, we need these course-of-life needs, and therein lies their objective importance. We need them whatever else we need. For example, it is sometimes said that whatever our chosen goals or tasks, we need our health, and so appropriate health care. But this claim is not strictly speaking true. For many of us, some of our goals, perhaps even those we feel most important to us, are not necessarily undermined by failing health or disability. Moreover, we can often adjust our goals—and presumably our levels of satisfaction— to fit better with our dysfunction or disability. Coping in this way does not necessarily diminish happiness or satisfaction in life.

Still, there is a clue here to a more plausible account: impairments of normal species functioning reduce the range of opportunity we have within which to construct life-plans and conceptions of the good we have a reasonable expectation of finding satisfying or happiness-producing. Moreover, if persons have a high-order interest in preserving the opportunity to revise their conceptions of the good through time, then they will have a pressing interest in maintaining normal species functioning by establishing institutions—such as health-care systems—which do just that. So the kinds of needs Braybrooke and McCloskey pick out by reference to normal species functioning are objectively important because they meet this high-order interest persons have in maintaining a normal range of opportunities. I shall try to refine this admittedly vague answer, but first I want to characterize health-care needs more specifically and show that they fit within this more general framework.

IV. HEALTH-CARE NEEDS

Disease and Health

To specify a notion of health-care needs, we need clear notions of health and disease. I shall begin with a narrow, if not uncontroversial, "biomedical" model of disease and health. The basic idea is that health is the absence of disease and diseases (I here include deformities and disabilities that result from trauma) are *deviations from the natural functional organization of a typical member of a species*.[12] The task of characterizing this natural functional organization falls to the biomedical sciences, which must include evolutionary theory since claims about the design of the species and its fitness to meeting biological goals underlie at least some of the relevant functional ascriptions. The task is the same for man and beast with two complications. For humans we require an account of the species-typical functions that permit us to pursue biological goals as social animals. So there must be a way of characterizing the species-typical apparatus underlying such functions as the acquisition of knowledge, linguistic communication, and social cooperation. Moreover, adding mental disease and health into the picture complicates the issue further, most particularly because we have a less well-developed theory of species typical mental functions and functional organization. The "biomedical" model clearly presupposes we can, in theory, supply the missing account and that a reasonable part of what we now take to be psychopathology would show up as diseases.[13]

The biomedical model has two controversial features. First, the deviations that play a role in the definition of disease are from species-typical functional organization. In contrast, some treat health as an idealized level of fully developed functioning, as in the WHO definition.[14] Others insist that the notion of disease is strictly normative and that diseases are deviations from socially preferred functional

12. The account here draws on a fine series of articles by Christopher Boorse; see "On the Distinction Between Disease and Illness," *Philosophy & Public Affairs* 5, no. 1 (Fall 1975): 49-68 and above, pp. 3-22; "What a Theory of Mental Health Should Be," *Journal of the Theory of Social Behavior* 6, no. 1: 61-84; "Health as a Theoretical Concept," *Philosophy of Science* 44 (1977): 542-573. See also Ruth Macklin, "Mental Health and Mental Illness: Some Problems of Definition and Concept Formation," *Philosophy of Science* 39, no. 3 (September 1972): 341-365.

13. Boorse, "What a Theory of Mental Health Should Be," p. 77.

14. Health is a state of complete physical, mental, and social well-being, and not merely the absence of disease or infirmity." From the Preamble to the Constitution of the World Health Organization. Adopted by the International Health Conference held in New York, 19 June-22 July 1946, and signed on 22 July 1946. *Off. Rec. Wld. Health Org.* 2, no. 100. See Daniel Callahan, "The WHO Definition of 'Health,'" *The Hastings Center Studies* 1, no. 3 (1973): 77-88.

norms.[15] Still, the WHO definition seems to conflate notions of health with those of general well-being, satisfaction, or happiness, over-medicalizing the domain of social philosophy. And, historical, arguments which show that "deviant" functioning—for example, "Drape-tomania" (the running-away disease of slaves) or masturbation—have been medicalized and viewed as diseases do not establish the strongly normative thesis that deviance from social norms of functioning constitutes disease. So I shall accept the first feature of the model, noting, of course, that the model does not exclude normative judgments *about* diseases, for example, about which are undesirable or which excuse us from normally criticizable behavior and justify our entering a "sick role." These judgments circumscribe the normative notion of illness or sickness, not the theoretically more basic notion of disease (which thus admittedly departs from looser ordinary usage).[16]

Second, pure forms of the biomedical model also involve a deeper claim, namely that species-normal functional organization can itself be characterized without invoking normative or value judgments. Here the debate turns on hard issues in the philosophy of biology.[17] Fortunately, these need not detain us since my discussion does not turn on so strong a claim. It is enough for my purposes if the line between disease and the absence of disease is, for the general run of cases, *uncontroversial* and ascertainable through publicly acceptable methods, for example, primarily those of the biomedical sciences. It will not matter if there is some relativization of what counts as a disease category to some features of social roles in a given society, and thus

15. See H. Tristram Engelhardt, Jr., "The Disease of Masturbation: Values and the Concept of Disease," *Bulletin of the History of Medicine* 48, no. 2 (Summer 1974): 234-248.

16. Boorse's critique of strongly normative views of disease is persuasive independently of some problematic features of his own account.

17. For example, we need an account of functional ascriptions in biology (see Boorse, "Wright on Functions," *Philosophical Review* 85, no. 1 [January 1976]: 70-86). More specifically, we need to be able to distinguish genetic variations from disease, and we must specify the range of environments taken as "natural" for the purpose of revealing dysfunction. The latter is critical to the second feature of the biomedical model: for example, what range of social roles and environments is included in the natural range? If we allow too much of the social environment, then racially discriminatory environments might make being of the wrong race a disease; if we disallow all socially created environments, then we seem not to be able to call dyslexia a disease (disability).

to some normative judgments, provided the core of the notion of species normal functioning is left intact. The model would still, I presume, count infertility as a disease, even though some or many individuals might prefer to be infertile and seek medical treatment to render themselves so. Similarly, unwanted pregnancy is not a disease. Again, dysfunctional noses are diseases, since noses have normal species functions and anatomy. If the dysfunction or deformity is serious, it might warrant treatment as an illness. But deviation of nasal anatomy from individual or social conceptions of beauty does not constitute disease.[18]

Thus the modified biomedical model still allows me to draw a fairly sharp line between uses of health-care services to prevent and treat diseases and uses to meet other social goals. The importance of such other goals may be different and may rest on other bases, for example, in the induced infertility or unwanted pregnancy cases. My intention is to show which principles of justice are relevant to distributing health-care services where we can take as fixed, primarily by nature, a generally uncontroversial baseline of species-normal functional organization. If important moral considerations enter at yet another level, to determine what counts as health and what disease, then the principles I discuss and these others must be reconciled, a task the biomedical model makes unnecessary at this stage and which I want to avoid here in any case. Of course, a complete theory, which I do not pursue, would presumably have to establish priorities among principles governing the meeting of health-care needs and principles for using health-care services to meet other social or individual goals, for example the termination of unwanted pregnancy or the upgrading of the beauty of the population.[19]

18. Anyone who doubts the appropriateness of treating some physiognomic deformities as serious diseases with strong claims on surgical resources should look at Frances C. MacGreggor's *After Plastic Surgery: Adaptation and Adjustment* (New York: Praeger, 1979). Even where there is no disease or deformity, there is nothing in the analysis I offer that precludes individuals or society from deciding to use health-care technology to make physiognomy conform to some standard of beauty. But such uses of health technology will not be justifiable as the fulfillment of health-care *needs*.

19. My account has the following bearing on the debate about Medicaid-funded abortions. Non-therapeutic abortions do not count as health-care needs, so *if* Medicaid has as its only function the meeting of the health-care needs

*Health-Care Needs
and Distributive Justice*

Though I have deliberately selected a rather narrow model of disease and health, at least by comparison to some fashionable construals, *health-care needs* emerge as a broad and diverse set. Health-care needs will be those things we need in order to maintain, restore, or provide functional equivalents (where possible) to, normal species functioning. They can be divided into:

(1) adequate nutrition, shelter
(2) sanitary, safe, unpolluted living and working conditions
(3) exercise, rest, and other features of healthy life-styles
(4) preventive, curative, and rehabilitative personal medical services
(5) non-medical personal (and social) support services

Of course, we do not tend to think of all these things as included among health-care needs, partly because we tend to think narrowly about personal medical services when we think about health care. But the list is not constructed to conform to our ordinary notion of health care but to point out a functional relation between quite diverse goods and services, and the various institutions responsible for delivering them.

Disease and Opportunity

The *normal opportunity range* for a given society will be the array of "life-plans" reasonable persons in it are likely to construct for themselves. The range is thus relative to key features of the society—its stage of historical development, its level of material wealth and technological development, and even important cultural facts about it. Facts about social organization, including the conception of justice regulating its basic institutions, will of course determine how that total normal range is distributed in the population. Nevertheless, that issue of distribution aside, normal species-typical functioning provides

---

of the poor, then we cannot argue for funding the abortions just like any other procedure. Their justifications will be different. But if Medicaid should serve other important goals, like ensuring that poor and well-off women can equally well control their bodies, then there is justification for funding abortions. There is also the worry that not funding them will contribute to other health problems induced by illegal abortions.

us with one clear parameter relevant to defining the normal opportunity range. Consequently, impairment of normal functioning through disease constitutes a fundamental restriction on individual opportunity relative to the normal opportunity range.

There are two important points to note about the normal opportunity range. Obviously some diseases constitute more serious curtailments of opportunity than others relative to a given range. But because normal ranges are society relative, the same disease in two societies may impair opportunity differently and so have their importance assessed differently. Thus the social importance of particular diseases is a notion we plausibly ought to relativize between societies, assuming for the moment that impairment of opportunity is a relevant consideration. Within a society, however, the normal opportunity-range abstracts from important individual differences in what might be called *effective opportunity*. From the perspective of an individual with a particular conception of the good (life plan or utility function), one who has developed certain skills and capacities needed to carry out chosen projects, *effective* opportunity range will be a subspace of the normal range. A college teacher whose career and recreational skills rely little on certain kinds of manual dexterity might find his effective opportunity diminished little compared to what a skilled laborer might find if disease impaired that dexterity. By appealing to the normal range I abstract from these differences in effective range, just as I avoid appeals directly to a person's conception of the good when I seek a measure for the social importance (for claims of justice) of health care needs.[20]

What emerges here is the suggestion that we use impairment of the normal opportunity range as a fairly crude measure of the relative importance of health-care needs at the macro level. In general, it will be more important to prevent, cure, or compensate for those disease conditions which involve a greater curtailment of normal opportunity range. Of course, impairment of normal species-functioning has another distinct effect. It can diminish satisfaction or happiness for an individual, as judged by that individual's conception of

20. One issue here is to avoid "hijacking" by past preferences which themselves define the effective range. Of course, effective range may be important in micro allocation decisions.

the good. Such effects are important at the micro level—for example, to individual decision-making about health-care utilization. But I am here seeking the appropriate framework within which to apply principles of justice to health care at the macro level. So we shall have to look further at considerations that weigh against appeals to satisfaction at the macro level.

V. Toward a Distributive Theory

Satisfaction and Narrower Measures of Well-Being

So far my discussion has been primarily descriptive, not normative. As Scanlon suggests, we do not in fact use a full-range satisfaction criterion of well-being when we assess the importance or urgency of individual claims on our resources. Rather, we treat as important only a narrow range of kinds of preferences. More specifically, preferences that bear on the fulfilment of certain kinds of needs are important components of this truncated scale of well-being. In a broad range of moral contexts, we give precedence to claims based on such needs, including health-care needs, over claims based on other kinds of preferences. The Braybrooke and McCloskey suggestion gives us a general characterization of this class of needs: deficiency with regard to them threatens normal species-functioning. More specifically, we can characterize health-care needs as things we need to maintain, restore, or compensate for the loss of, normal species-functioning. Since serious impairments of normal functioning diminish our capacities and abilities, they impair individual opportunity range relative to the range normal for our society. If we suppose people have an interest in maintaining a fair and roughly equal opportunity range, we can give at least a plausible *explanation* why they think health-care needs are special and important (which is not to say we actually do distribute them accordingly).

In what follows, I shall urge a normative claim: we ought to subsume health care under a principle of justice guaranteeing fair equality of opportunity. Actually, since I cannot here defend such a general principle without going too deeply into the general theory of distributive justice, I shall urge a weaker claim: *if* an acceptable theory of justice includes a principle providing for fair equality of opportunity, then health-care institutions should be among those governed by it. Indeed, I shall sketch briefly how one general theory, Rawls' theory of justice as fairness, might be extended in this way to provide a distributive theory for health care. *But my account does not presuppose the acceptability of Rawls' theory.* If a rule or ideal code-utilitarianism, or some other theory, establishes a fair equality of opportunity principle, my account will probably be compatible with it (though some of the argument that follows may not be).

In order to introduce some issues relevant to extending Rawls' theory, I want to consider an issue we have thus far left hanging. *Should* we, for purposes of justice, use the objective, truncated scale of well-being we happen to use rather than a full-range satisfaction scale? Clearly, this too is a general question that takes us beyond the scope of this essay. Moreover, it is unlikely that we could establish conclusively a case against the satisfaction scale by considering the health care context alone. For example, a utilitarian proponent of a satisfaction of enjoyment scale might claim that the general tendencies of different diseases to diminish satisfaction provides, at worst, a rough equivalent to the "impairment of opportunity" criterion I am proposing.[21] Still, it is worth suggesting some of the considerations that weigh against the use of a satisfaction scale.

We can begin by pointing to a special case where our moral judgment would incline us against using a satisfaction scale, namely the case of "social hijacking" by persons with expensive tastes.[22] Suppose we judge how well-off someone is by reference to the full range of individual preferences in a satisfaction scale. Suppose further that moderate people adjust their tastes and preferences so that they have a reasonable chance of being satisfied with their share of social goods. Other more extravagant people form exotic and expensive tastes, even though they have comparable shares to the moderates, and, because their preferences are very strong, they are desperately unhappy when these tastes are not satisfied. Assume we can agree intersubjectively that the extravagants are less satisfied. Then if

21. Presumably, he must also claim that we improve satisfaction more by treating and preventing disease than by finding ways to encourage people to adjust to their conditions by reordering their preference curves.

22. I draw on Rawls' unpublished lecture, "Responsibility for Ends," in the following three paragraphs.

we are interested in maximizing—or even equalizing—satisfaction, extravagants seem to have a greater claim or further distributions of social resources than moderates. But something seems clearly unjust if we deny the moderates equal claims on further distributions just because they have been modest in forming their tastes. With regard to tastes and preferences that *could have been otherwise* had the extravagants chosen differently, it seems reasonable to hold them *responsible* for their own low level of satisfaction.[23]

A more general division of responsibility is suggested by this hijacking case. Rawls urges that we hold *society* responsible for guaranteeing the individual a fair share of basic liberties, opportunity, and all-purpose means, like income and wealth, needed for pursuing individual conceptions of the good. But the *individual* is responsible for choosing his ends in such a way that he has a reasonable chance of satisfying them under such just arrangements.[24] Consequently, the special features of an individual's conception of the good—here his extravagant tastes and resulting dissatisfaction—do not give rise to any special claims of justice on social resources. This suggestion about a division of responsibility is really a claim about the *scope* of theories of justice: just arrangements are supposed to guarantee individuals a reasonable share of certain basic social goods which constitute the relevant—truncated—scale of well-being for purposes of justice. The immediate object of justice is not, then, happiness or the satisfaction of desires, though just institutions provide individuals with an acceptable framework within which they can seek happiness and pursue their interests. But individuals remain responsible for the choice of their ends, so there is no injustice in not having sufficient means to reach extravagant ends.

Obviously, a full defense of this claim about the scope of justice and the social division of responsibility, and thus about the reasons

23. Here again the utilitarian proponent of the satisfaction scale may issue a typical promissory note, assuring us that maximizing satisfaction overall requires institutional arrangements that act to minimize social hijacking.

24. The division presupposes, as Rawls points out in response to Scanlon, that people have the ability and know they have the responsibility to adjust their desires in view of their fair shares of (primary) social goods. See Scanlon, "Preference and Urgency," pp. 665-666.

for using a truncated scale of well-being, cannot rest on isolated intuitions about cases like the hijacking one. In Rawls' case, a full argument involves the claim that adopting a satisfaction scale commits
us to an unacceptable view of persons as mere "containers" for satisfaction, one that departs significantly from our moral practice.[25] Because I cannot pursue these issues here, beyond suggesting there are
problems with a satisfaction scale, I am content to show there is a
systematic, plausible alternative to using a satisfaction scale (and
ultimately to utilitarianism) whose acceptability depends on more
general issues. Consequently I stick with my weaker, conditional
claim above.

Rawls' argument for a truncated scale is, of course, for a specific
scale, one composed of his primary social goods. But my talk about
a truncated scale has focused on talk about certain basic needs, in
particular, things we need to maintain species-typical normal functioning. Health-care needs are paradigmatic among these. The task
that remains is to fit the two scales together. My analysis of the relation between disease and normal opportunity range provides the
key to doing that.

Extending Rawls' Theory to Health Care

Rawls' *index of primary social goods*—his truncated scale of well-
being used in the contract—includes five types of social goods: (a)
a set of basic liberties; (b) freedom of movement and choice of oc-
cupations against a background of diverse opportunities; (c) powers
and prerogatives of office; (d) income and wealth; (e) the social
bases of self-respect. Actually, Rawls uses two simplifying assumptions when using the index to assess how well-off (representative)

25. Satisfaction scales leave us no basis for not wanting to *be* whatever
person, construed as a set of preferences, has higher satisfaction. To borrow
Bernard Williams' term, they leave us with no basis for insisting on the *integrity*
of persons. See Rawls, "Responsibility for Ends." The view that issues here turn
in a fundamental way on the nature of persons is pursued in Derek Parfit, "Later
Selves and Moral Principles," *Philosophy and Personal Relations*, ed. Alan
Montefiore (London: Routledge & Kegan Paul, 1973): 137-169; Rawls, "Independence of Moral Theory," *Proceedings and Addresses of the American Philosophical Association*, 48 (1974-1975): 5-22; and Daniels, "Moral Theory and the
Plasticity of Persons," *Monist* 62, no. 3 (July 1979): 265-287.

individuals are. First, income and wealth are used as approximations
to the whole index. Thus the two principles of justice[26] require basic
structures to maximize the long term expectations of the least advan-
taged, estimated by their income and wealth, given fixed background
institutions that guarantee equal basic liberties and fair equality of
opportunity. More importantly for our purposes, the theory is *idealized*
to apply to individuals who are "normal, active and fully cooperating
members of society over the course of a complete life."[27] There is no
distributive theory for health care because no one is sick.

This simplification seems to put Rawls' index at odds with the thrust
of my earlier discussion, for the truncated scale of well-being we in
fact use includes needs for health care. The primary goods seem to
be *too truncated* a scale, once we drop the idealizing assumption.
People with equal indices will not be equally well-off once we allow
them to differ in health-care needs. Moreover, we cannot simply dismiss these needs as irrelevant to questions of justice, as we did certain tastes and preferences. But if we simply build another entry into
the index, we raise special issues about how to arrive at an approxi-
mate weighting of the index items.[28] Similarly, if we treat health-
care services as a specially important primary social good, we
abandon the useful generality of the notion of a primary social good.
Moreover, we risk generating a long list of such goods, one to meet
each important need.[29] Finally, as I argued earlier in answer to Fried's
proposal about insurance schemes, we cannot just finesse the question whether there are special issues of justice in the distribution of
health care by assuming fair shares of primary goods will be used
in part to buy decent health-care insurance. A constraint on the
adequacy of those shares is that they permit one to buy reasonable

26. See *A Theory of Justice* (Cambridge: Harvard, 1971), p. 302.

27. Rawls, "Responsibility for Ends."

28. Some weighting problems will have to be faced anyway; see my "Rights
to Health Care" for further discussion. Also see Kenneth Arrow, "Some Ordinalist
Utilitarian Notes on Rawls's Theory of Justice," *Journal of Philosophy* 70, no.
9 (1973); 245-263. Also see Joshua Cohen, "Studies in Political Philosophy,"
Ph.D. diss. (Harvard University, 1978), Part III and Appendices.

29. See Ronald Greene, "Health Care and Justice in Contract Theory Perspective," in *Ethics & Health Policy*, ed. Robert Veatch and Roy Branson (Cambridge,
MA: Ballinger, 1976), pp. 111-126.

protection—so we must already know what justice requires by way of reasonable health care.

The most promising strategy for extending Rawls' theory without tampering with useful assumptions about the index of primary goods simply includes health-care institutions among the background institutions involved in providing for fair equality of opportunity.[30] Once we note the special connection of normal species functioning to the opportunity range open to an individual, this strategy seems the natural way to extend Rawls' view that *the subject* of theories of social justice are the *basic institutions* which provide a framework of liberties and opportunities within which individuals can use fair income-shares to pursue their own conceptions of the good. Insofar as meeting health-care needs has an important effect on the distribution of health, and more to the point, on the distribution of opportunity, the health-care institutions are plausibly included on the list of basic institutions a fair equality of opportunity principle should regulate.[31]

Including health-care institutions among those which are to protect fair equality of opportunity is compatible with the central intuitions behind wanting to guarantee such opportunity in the first place. Rawls is primarily concerned with *the opportunity to pursue careers*—jobs and offices—that have various benefits attached to them. So equality of opportunity is *strategically* important: a person's well being will

30. The primary social goods themselves remain general and abstract properties of social arrangements—basic liberties, opportunities, and certain all-purpose exchangeable means (income and wealth). We can still simplify matters in using the index by looking solely at income and wealth—assuming a background of equal basic liberties and fair equality of opportunity. Health care is not a primary social good—neither are food, clothing, shelter, or other basic needs. The presumption is that the latter will be adequately provided for from fair shares of income and wealth. The special importance and unequal distribution of health-care needs, like educational needs, are acknowledged by their connection to other institutions that provide for fair equality of opportunity. But opportunity, not health care or education, is the primary social good.

31. Here I shift emphasis from Rawls when he remarks that health is a *natural* as opposed to *social* primary good because its possession is less influenced by basic institutions. See *A Theory of Justice*, p. 62. Moreover, it seems to follow that where health care is generally inefficacious—say, in earlier centuries—it loses its status as a special concern of justice and the "caring" it offers may more properly be viewed as a concern of charity.

be measured for the most part by the primary goods that accompany placement in such jobs and offices.[32] Rawls argues it is not enough simply to eliminate formal or legal barriers to persons seeking such jobs—for example, race, class, ethnic, or sex barriers. Rather, positive steps should be taken to enhance the opportunity of those disadvantaged by such social factors as family background.[33] The point is that none of us *deserves* the advantages conferred by accidents of birth—either the genetic or social advantages. These advantages from the "natural lottery" are morally arbitrary, and to let them determine individual opportunity—and reward and success in life—is to confer arbitrariness on the outcomes. So positive steps, for example, through the educational system, are to be taken to provide fair equality of opportunity.[34]

But if it is important to use resources to counter the advantages in opportunity some get in the natural lottery, it is equally important to use resources to counter the natural disadvantages induced by disease (and since class-differentiated social conditions contribute significantly to the etiology of disease, we are reminded disease is not just a product of the natural component of the lottery). But this does not mean we are committed to the futile goal of eliminating all natural differences between persons. Health care has as its goal normal functioning and so concentrates on a specific class of obvious disadvantages and tries to eliminate them. That is its *limited* contribution to guaranteeing fair equality of opportunity.

The approach taken here allows us to draw some interesting parallels between education and health care, for both are strategically important contributors to fair equality of opportunity. Both address needs which are not equally distributed between individuals. Various social

32. The ways in which disease affects normal opportunity range are more extensive than the ways in which it affects opportunity to pursue careers, a point I return to later.

33. Of course, the effects of family background cannot all be eliminated. See *A Theory of Justice*, p. 74.

34. Rawls allows individual differences in talents and abilities to remain relevant to issues of job placement, for example, through their effects on productivity. So fair equality of opportunity does not mean that individual differences no longer confer advantages. Advantages are constrained by the difference principle. See my "Merit and Meritocracy," *Philosophy & Public Affairs* 7, no. 3 (Spring 1978): 206-223.

factors, such as race, class, and family background, may produce special learning needs; so too may natural factors, such as the broad class of learning disabilities. To the extent that education is aimed at providing fair equality of opportunity, special provision must be made to meet these special needs. Here educational needs, like health care needs, differ from other basic needs, such as the need for food and clothing, which are more equally distributed between persons. The combination of unequal distribution and the great strategic importance of the opportunity to have health care and education puts these needs in a separate category from those basic needs we can expect people to purchase from their fair-income shares.

It is worth noting another point of fit between my analysis and Rawls' theory. In Rawls' contract situation, a "thick" veil of ignorance is imposed on contractors choosing basic principles of justice: they do not know their abilities, talents, place in society, or historical period. In selecting principles to govern health-care resource-allocation decisions, we need a thinner veil, for we must know about some features of the society, for example, its resource limitations. Still, using the normal opportunity range and not just the effective range as the baseline has the effect of imposing a plausibly thinned veil. It reflects basic facts about the society but keeps facts about individuals' particular ends from unduly influencing social decisions. Ultimately, defense of a veil depends on the theory of the person underlying the account. The intuition here is that persons are not defined by a particular set of interests but are free to revise their life plans. Consequently, they have an interest in maintaining conditions under which they can revise such plans, which makes the normal range a plausible reference point.

Subsuming health-care institutions under the opportunity principle can be viewed as a way of keeping the system as close as possible to the original idealization under which Rawls' theory was constructed, namely, that we are concerned with normal, fully functioning persons with a complete life span. An important set of institutions can thus be viewed as a first defense of the idealization: they act to minimize the likelihood of departures from the normality assumption. Included here are institutions which provide for public health, environmental cleanliness, preventive personal medical services, occupational health and safety, food and drug protection, nutritional education, and educational and incentive measures to promote individual responsibility for healthy life styles. A second layer of institutions corrects departures from the idealization. It includes those which deliver personal medical and rehabilitative services that restore normal functioning. A third layer attempts, where feasible, to maintain persons in a way that is as close as possible to the idealization. Institutions involved with more extended medical and social support services for the (moderately) chronically ill and disabled and the frail elderly would fit here. Finally, a fourth layer involves health care and related social services for those who can in no way be brought closer to the idealization. Terminal care and care for the seriously mentally and physically disabled fit here, but they raise serious issues which may not just be issues of justice. Indeed, by the time we get to the fourth layer moral virtues other than justice become prominent.

VI. WORRIES AND QUALIFICATIONS

I would like to address two kinds of worries that arise in response to the approach to equality of opportunity that I have been sketching, though no doubt there are others.[35] One is that the account cannot be *exhaustive* of distributive issues in health care—the connection to opportunity is but one consideration among many. A second worry is that the appeal to opportunity is not a *useable* one—it commits us to too much or fails to tell us what we are committed to. Both worries emphasize the degree to which my account is programmatic.

35. For example, appeals to equality of opportunity have historically played a conservative, deceptive role, blinding people to the injustice of class and race inequalities in rewards. Historically, appeals to the ideal of equal opportunity have implicitly justified strong competitive individual relations. More concretely, we often find institutions, like the United States educational system, praised as embodying (at least approximately) that ideal, whereas there is strong evidence the system functions primarily to replicate class inequalities. See my "IQ, Heritability and Human Nature" in *Proceedings of the Philosophy of Science Association, 1974*, ed. R. S. Cohen (Dordrecht: Reidel, 1976), pp. 143-180; and, with J. Cronin, A. Krock, and R. Webber, "Race, Class and Intelligence: A Critical Look at the IQ Controversy," *International Journal of Mental Health* 3, no. 4: 46-123; and S. Bowles and H. Gintis, *Schooling in Capitalist America* (New York: Basic Books, 1976).

One way to put the first worry is that my account makes the "specialness" of health care rest on quite abstract considerations. After all, when we reflect on the importance of health-care needs, many other factors than their effects on opportunity come to mind. Some might say health care in a direct and simple way reduces pain and suffering—and no fancy analysis of opportunity is needed to show why people value reducing them. Still, much health care affects quality of life in other ways, so the benefit of reducing pain and suffering is not general enough for our purposes. Moreover, some suffering, for example, some emotional suffering, though a cause for concern, does not obviously become a concern of justice. Others may point to psychological or cultural bases for our viewing health care as special, for example, disease reminds us of the fragility of life and the limits of human existence. But even if this point is relevant to sociological or psychological explanations of the importance some of us attribute to some kinds of health care, I have been attempting a different kind of analysis, one that can be used to justify and not just explain the importance attached to health care. So I have abstracted a central *function* of health care, the maintenance of species-typical function, and noted its central *effect* on opportunity. As a result, we are in a better position to frame distributive principles that account for the special way we treat health care because we can now say what kind of a social good health-care is, namely one that maintains normal opportunity range. My analysis, while not exhaustive, focuses on that general benefit which is most relevant from the point of view of distributive justice.

Still, this qualification does not settle the first worry, which can be raised in another way. Within the confines of Rawls' theory, fair equality of opportunity—and Rawls' principle guaranteeing it—is concerned solely with access to jobs and offices. In contrast, my notion of normal opportunity range is far broader. To be sure, the narrower notion, whatever its problems, is far clearer than the broader one. But if we stick with the narrower one, we immediately import a strong age bias into our distributive theory. The opportunity of the elderly to enter jobs or offices is not impaired by disease since they are beyond, as the crass phrase goes, their "productive" years. Thus fair equality of opportunity narrowly construed seems open to one of the standard objections raised against "productivity" measures of the value of life.[36]

There are two ways to respond to this problem while still adhering to the narrower construal of opportunity. One is to admit that equality of opportunity is only one among several considerations that bear on the justice of health-care distribution. Still, even on this view, it is an important consideration with broad implications for health care delivery. Fleshing out this response would require showing how the opportunity principle fits with these other considerations. A stronger response is to claim that the domain of basic considerations of *justice* regarding health care is exhausted by the equal opportunity principle. Other moral considerations may bear on distribution, but claims of justice will be based on the narrowly construed opportunity principle. This response bites the bullet about the age effect.

If we turn to the broader construal of equality of opportunity, using the notion of normal opportunity range, the problem reemerges, as do the weaker and stronger responses, but there may be more flexibility. The problem reemerges because it might seem that the young will always suffer greater impairment of opportunity than the elderly if health-care needs are not met. But a further alternative suggests itself: it may be possible to make the normal opportunity range relative to age. On this view, for each age (stage of life) there is a normal opportunity range, but it reflects basic facts about the life cycle and a society's responses to it. Consequently, diseases may have different effects on the young and elderly and their importance will be assessed differently.[37] This approach may avoid the most serious objections about age-bias. It still leaves open the weak claim that the opportunity principle is only one consideration among

36. See E. J. Mishan, "Evaluation of Life and Limb: a Theoretical Approach," *Journal of Political Economy*, 79, no. 4 (1971): 687-705; Jan Paul Acton, "Measuring the Monetary Value of Life Saving Programs," *Law and Contemporary Problems* 40, no. 4 (Autumn 1976): 46-72; Michael Bayles, "The Price of Life," *Ethics* 89, no. 1 (October 1978): 20-34.

37. It would be interesting to know if this age-relativized opportunity range yields results similar to that achieved by the Rawlsian device of a veil. If people who do not know their age are asked to design a system of health-care delivery for the society they will be in, they would presumably budget their resources in a fashion that takes the special features of each stage of the life cycle into account and gives each stage a reasonable claim on resources.

many or the stronger claim that it circumscribes the scope of basic claims of justice. The stronger claim may seem more plausible since the opportunity principle has broader scope on this construal. But employing the broader construal brings with it other serious problems: do arguments which establish the priority of fair equality of opportunity on the narrow construal with its competitive aspect extend to the broader notion? These issues and alternatives require more careful discussion than they can be given here.

The second worry, about what commitments the appeal to equal opportunity generates, also has several sources. Certain "hard" cases raise the issue sharply. What does asking for the restoration of normal opportunity range mean for the terminally ill, on whom we lavish exotic life-prolonging technology, or for the severely mentally retarded? We are not required to pour all our resources into the worst cases, for that would undermine our ability to protect the opportunity of many others. But I am not sure what the approach requires here, if it delivers an answer at all. Similarly, the approach provides little help with another sort of hard case, the resource allocation decisions in which we must choose between services which remove serious impairments of opportunity for a few people and those which remove significant but less serious impairments from many. But these shortcomings are not special to the approach I sketch: distributive theories generally founder on such cases. It seems reasonable to test my approach first in the cases where we have a better understanding of what kind of health care is owed. In any case, I do not rule out here the strong response sketched earlier to the worry about exhaustiveness, namely that our problem with at least the first kind of hard case derives from the fact that it takes us beyond the domain of justice into other considerations of right.

The second worry also has more fundamental sources. Suppose supplying a car to everyone who cannot afford one would do more to remove individual impairments of normal opportunity range than supplying certain health care services to those who need them. Does the opportunity approach commit us now to supply cars instead of treatments?[38] The example is an instance of a far more general prob-

38. Using medical technology to enhance normal capacities or functions—say strength or vision—makes the problem easier: the burden of proof is on

lem, namely, that socioeconomic (and other) inequalities affect opportunity (broadly or narrowly construed), not just the health-care and educational needs we have picked out as strategically important. But my approach does not require me to deny that certain inequalities in wealth and income may conflict with fair equality of opportunity and that guaranteeing fair equality of opportunity may thus constrain acceptable inequalities in these goods. Rather, my approach rests on the calculation that certain institutions meet needs which quite generally have a central impact on opportunity range and which should therefore be governed directly by the opportunity principle.

Finally, the second worry can be traced to the fear that health-care needs are so *expansive* (and expensive), given the advance of technology, that they create a bottomless pit. Fried, for example, argues that recognizing individual right claims to the satisfaction of health-care needs would force society to forgo realizing other social goals. He cautions we would end up worshipping the opportunity to pursue our goals but having to forgo the pursuit. Here we have the other form of the social hijacking argument, hijacking by needs rather than preferences.[39]

Two points can be offered in response to Fried's version of the second worry. First, the narrow model I have given of health-care needs excludes some of the kinds of cases Fried uses to demonstrate the threat of the bottomless pit. Thus Fried's example of retarding the effects of normal aging does not emerge as a *need* on my analysis, since normal aging does not involve a departure from normal species functioning. Such uses of health-care technology may be thought important in a particular society. Then, arguments about the relative merits of this use of scarce resources may be advanced. But such arguments would not rest on claims about basic health-care needs and thus may have different justificatory force. Still, technology does expand the ways (and costs) we have of meeting

---

proposals that give priority to altering the normal opportunity range rather than protecting individuals whose normal range is compromised.

39. See Fried, *Right and Wrong*, chap. 5. The problem also worries Braybrooke, "Let Needs Diminish."

genuine health care needs. So my account of needs at best reduces
but does not eliminate Fried's worry.

Second, there is a difference between Fried's account of individual
rights and entitlements and the one I am assuming here (which is
quite Rawlsian). Fried is worried that if we posit a fundamental
individual right to have needs satisfied, no other social goals will be
able to override the right claims to all health care needs.[10] But no such
fundamental right is *directly* posited on the view I have sketched.
Rather, the particular rights and entitlements of individuals to have
certain needs met are specified only *indirectly*, as a result of the basic
health-care institutions acting in accord with the general principle
governing opportunity. Deciding which needs are to be met and
what resources are to be devoted to doing so requires careful moral
judgment. The various institutions which affect opportunity must be
weighed against each other. Similarly, the resources required to provide for fair equality of opportunity must be weighed against what
is needed to provide for other important social institutions. Clearly,
health-care institutions capable of protecting opportunity can be
maintained only in societies whose productive capacities they do
not undermine. The bugaboo of the bottomless pit is less threatening
in the context of such a theory. The price paid is that we are less
clear—in general and abstracting from the application of the theory
to a given society—just what the individual claim comes to. The price
is worth paying.

These worries emphasize the sense in which my account is sketchy
and programmatic. It is worth a reminder that my account is incomplete in other ways. I have not argued that opportunity-based
considerations are the only ones that should bear on the design of
health care systems. Other important social goals—some protected by
right claims or other claims of need—may require the use of health-
care technology. I have not considered when, if ever, these needs or
rights take precedence over other wants and preferences or over
some health-care needs.[41] Similarly, there is the question whether the
demand for equality in health care extends beyond some decent

40. It is not clear to me how much Fried's side-constraints resemble Nozick's.
41. See fn. 19 above.

adequate minimum—which we may suppose is defined by reference
to fair equality of opportunity. Should those health-care services not
considered basic be allowed to operate on a market basis? Should we
insist on equality even here? These issues are not addressed by my
analysis.[42]

Finally, my account is incomplete because I have concentrated
on social obligations to maintain and restore health and have ignored
individual responsibility to do so. But there is substantial evidence
that individuals can do much to avoid incurring risks to their health—
by avoiding smoking, excess alcohol, and certain foods, and by get-
ting adequate exercise and rest. Now, nothing in my approach is incompatible with encouraging people to adopt healthy lifestyles. The
harder issue, however, is deciding how to distribute the burdens that
result when people "voluntarily" incur extra risks and swell the costs
of health care by doing so (by over 10 percent, on some estimates).
After all, the consequences of such behavior cannot be easily dismissed as the arbitrary outcome of the natural lottery. Should smokers
be forced to pay higher insurance premiums or special health-care
taxes? I do not believe my account forces us to ignore the source of
health-care risks in assigning such burdens. But at this point little
more can be said because much here depends on very specific details
of social history. In the United States, government subsidies of the
tobacco industry, the legality of cigarette advertising, the legality of
smoking in public places, and special subculture pressures on key
groups (for example, teenagers) all undermine the view that we have
clear-cut cases of informed, individual decision-making for which
individuals must be held fully accountable.

VII. APPLICATIONS

The account of health-care needs sketched here has a number of
implications of interest to health planners. Here I can only note

42. Except where conditions of extensive scarcity leave basic health-care
needs unmet and so no room for less important uses of health care services,
or except where the existence of a market-based health-care system threatens
the ability of the basic system to deliver its important product.

some of them and set aside the many difficulties that face drawing implications from ideal theory for non-ideal settings.[43]

Access

My account is compatible with (but does not imply) a multi-tiered health-care system. The basic tier would include health-care services that meet important health-care needs, defined by reference to their effects on opportunity. Other tiers would include services that meet less important health-care needs or other preferences. However the upper tiers are to be financed—through cost-sharing, at full-price, at "zero" price—[44] there should be no obstacles, financial, racial, sexual, or geographical to *initial access* to the system as a whole.

The equality of initial access derives from basic facts about the sociology and epistemology of the determination of health-care needs.[45] The "felt needs" of patients are (unreliable) initial indicators of real health care needs. Financial and geographical barriers to initial access—say to primary care—compel people to make their own determinations of the importance of their symptoms. Of course, every system requires some patient self-assessment, but financial and geographical barriers impose different burdens in such assessment on particular groups. Indeed, where sociological barriers exist to people utilizing services, positive steps are needed (in the schools, at work, in neighborhoods) to make sure unmet needs are detected.

It is sometimes argued that the difficult access problems are ones deriving from geographical barriers and the maldistribution of physicians within specialties. In the United States, it is often argued that achieving more equitable distribution of health care providers

43. I discuss these difficulties in "Conflicting Objectives and the Priorities Problem," in Peter Brown, Conrad Johnson, and Paul Vernier, eds., *Income Support: Conceptual and Policy Issues* (Totowa, N.J.: Rowman and Littlefield, 1981). My *Justice and Health Care Delivery* develops some applications in detail.

44. The strongest objections to such mixed systems is that the upper tier competes for resources with the lower tiers. See Claudine McCreadie, "Rawlsian Justice and the Financing of the National Health Service," *Journal of Social Policy* 5, no. 2 (1976): 113-131.

45. See Avedis Donabedian, *Aspects of Medical Care Administration* (Cambridge: Harvard, 1973).

would unduly constrain physician liberties. It is important to see that no fundamental liberties need be violated. Suppose that the basic tier of a health-care system is redistributively financed through a national health insurance scheme that eliminates financial barriers, that no alternative insurance for the basic tier is allowed, and that there is central planning of resource allocation to guarantee needs are met. To achieve a more equitable distribution of physicians, planners *license those eligible for reimbursement* in a given health-planning region according to some reasonable formula involving physician-patient ratios.[46] Additional providers might practice in an area, but they would be without benefit of third-party payments for all services in the basic tier (or for other tiers if the national insurance scheme is more comprehensive). Most providers would follow the reimbursement dollar and practice where they are most needed.

Far from violating basic liberties, the scheme merely puts physicians in the same relation to market constraints on job availability that face most other workers and professionals. A college professor cannot simply decide there are people to be taught in Scarsdale or Chevy Chase or Shaker Heights; he must accept what jobs are available within universities, wherever they are. Of course, he is "free" to ignore the market, but then he may not be able to teach. Similarly, managers and many types of workers face the need to locate themselves where there is need for their skills. So the physician's sacrifice of liberty under the scheme (or variants on it, including a National Health Service) is merely the imposition of a burden already faced by much of the working population. Indeed, the scheme does not change in principle the forces that already motivate physicians; it merely shifts where it is profitable for some physicians to practice. The appearance that there is an enshrined liberty under attack is the legacy of an historical accident, one more visible in the United States than elsewhere, namely, that physicians have been more independent of institutional settings for the delivery of their skills than many other

46. I ignore the crudeness of such measures. For fuller discussion of these manpower distribution issues see my "What is the Obligation of the Medical Profession in the Distribution of Health Care?" presented to the Conference on Health Care and Human Rights, University of Cincinnati Medical Center, 6 March 1980.

workers, and even than physicians in other countries. But this too shall pass.

Resource Allocation

My account of health-care needs and their connection to fair equality of opportunity has a number of implications for resource-allocation issues. I have already noted that we get an important distinction between the use of health-care services to meet health-care needs and their use to meet other wants and preferences. The tie of health-care needs to opportunity makes the former use special and important in a way not true of the latter. Moreover, we get a crude criterion—impact on normal opportunity range—for distinguishing the importance of different health-care needs, though I have also noted how far short this falls of being a solution to many hard allocation questions. Three further implications are worth noting here.

There has been much debate about whether the United States' health-care system overemphasizes acute therapeutic services as opposed to preventive and public health measures. Sometimes the argument focuses on the relative efficacy and cost of preventive, as opposed to acute, services. My account suggests there is also an important issue of distributive justice here. Suppose a system is heavily weighted toward acute interventions, yet it provides equal access to its services. Thus anyone with severe respiratory ailments—black lung, brown lung, asbestosis, emphysema, and so on—is given adequate and comprehensive services as needed. Does the system meet the demands of equity? Not if they are determined by the approach of fair equality of opportunity. The point is that people are differentially at risk of contracting such diseases because of work and living conditions. Efficacy aside, preventive measures have distinct distributive implications from acute measures. The opportunity approach requires we attend to both.

My account points to another allocational inequity. One important function of health-care services, here personal medical services, is to restore handicapping dysfunctions, for example, of vision, mobility, and so on. The medical goal is to cure the diseased organ or limb where possible. Where cure is impossible, we try to make function as normal as possible, through corrective lenses or prosthesis and rehabilitative therapy. But where restoration of function is beyond the ability of medicine per se, we begin to enter another area of services, non-medical social support (we move from (4) to (5) on the list of health-care needs in Section IV). Such support services provide the blind person with the closest he can get to the functional equivalent of vision—for example, he is taught how to navigate, provided with a seeing-eye dog, taught braille, and so on. From the point of view of their impact on opportunity, medical services and social support services that meet health-care needs have the same rationale and are equally important. Yet, for various reasons, probably having to do with the profitability and glamor of personal medical service and careers in them as compared to services for the handicapped, our society has taken only slow and halting steps to meet the health-care needs of those with permanent disabilities. These are matters of justice, not charity; we are not facing conditions of scarcity so severe that these steps to provide equality of opportunity must be forgone in favor of more pressing needs. The point also has implications for the problem of long term care for the frail elderly, but I cannot develop them here.

A final implication of the account raises a different set of issues, namely, how to reconcile the demands of justice with certain traditional views of a physician's obligation to his patients. The traditional view is that the physician's direct responsibility is to the well-being of his patients, that (with their consent) he is to do everything in his power to preserve their lives and well-being. One effect of leaving all resource-allocation decisions in this way to the micro-level decisions of physicians and patients, especially where third-party payment schemes mean little or no rationing by price, is that cost-ineffective utilization results. In the current cost-conscious climate, there is pressure to make physicians see themselves as responsible for introducing economic considerations into their utilization decisions. But the issue raised here goes beyond cost-effectiveness. My account suggests that there are important resource-allocation priorities that derive from considerations of justice. In a context of moderate scarcity, this suggests it is not possible for physicians to see as their ideal the maximization of the quality of care they deliver regardless of cost: pursuing that ideal upsets resource-allocation priorities determined by the opportunity principle. Considerations of justice challenge the traditional (perhaps mythical) view that physicians can act as the unrestrained agents of their patients. The remaining task, which I pursue elsewhere, is to show at what level the constraints should be imposed so as to disturb as little as possible of what is valuable about the traditional view of physician responsibility.[47]

These remarks on applications are frustratingly brief, and fuller development of them is required if we are to assess the practical import of the account I offer. Nevertheless, I think the account offers enough that it is attractive at the theoretical level to warrant further development of its practical implications.

47. See Avedis Donabedian "The Quality of Medical Care: A Concept in Search of a Definition," *Journal of Family Practice* 9, no. 2 (1979): 277-284; and Daniels, "Cost-Effectiveness and Patient Welfare," in Marc Basson, ed., *Rights and Responsibilities in Modern Medicine* (New York: Alan R. Liss, 1981), pp. 159-170.

Research for this paper was supported by Grant Number HS03097 from the National Center for Health Services Research, OASH, and by a Tufts Sabbatical Leave. I am also indebted to the Commonwealth Fund, which sponsored a seminar on this material at Brown University. Earlier drafts benefited from presentations to the Hastings Center Institute project on Ethics and Health Policy (funded by the Kaiser Foundation), a NCHSR staff seminar, and colloquia at Tufts, NYU Medical Center, University of Michigan, and University of Georgia. Helpful comments were provided by Ronald Bayer, Hugo Bedau, Richard Brandt, Dan Brock, Arthur Caplan, Josh Cohen, Allen Gibbard, Ruth Macklin, Carola Mone, John Rawls, Daniel Wikler, and the Editors of *Philosophy & Public Affairs*. This essay is excerpted from my *Justice and Health Care Delivery*, Cambridge University Press, in preparation.

LOREN E. LOMASKY Medical Progress and
National Health Care

An individual's access to medical care should not be determined exclusively by his ability to pay the going price. From this starting point, alternatives beckon. One is the traditional system of health-care delivery within which eleemosynary and religious institutions are prominent in providing medical services to those unable to pay. Before the emergence of modern medicine the poor could not expect treatment equivalent to that received by the rich, but this was a general disability of poverty, not specifically a problem of medical access. Indeed, in an era when health care had little positive correlation with health outcomes and hospitals were chiefly places where one went to die, inequities in the provision of medical services were among the least of the burdens borne by the poor.

Medical Progress and the "Right" to Health Care

The ability of medicine to produce favorable results has increased exponentially in this century. At the same time, for understandable reasons, dissatisfaction with the traditional model has also increased. It is criticized as being too haphazard and arbitrary. More fundamentally, it is argued that medical care is a good to which individuals have a right, and that it ought to be distributed impartially in line with the criterion: to each according to his need.[1] Medical care is not sim-

1. Variations on this theme abound. See Gene Outka, "Social Justice and Equal Access to Health Care," *Journal of Religious Ethics* 2 (1974): 11-32; Anne R. Somers and Herman M. Somers, "The Organization and Financing of

ply one consumer good among others; because it bears so directly on life itself as well as the ability to lead a good life, medical care cannot be left to the vagaries of the market.

But this argument is met with a counterargument that also emphasizes the role of rights. Medical services are, after all, not endowments provided cost-free by a bountiful nature. Rather, they are made available in finite quantities by individuals who must expend effort to produce them. The state can enforce equity in the delivery of these services only by coercing service providers, taxpayers and would-be recipients. State-controlled health care is thus founded on widespread rights violations.[2]

When right contends with right, the heroic seek victory, the wary hunt for accommodation. It is wariness that will be pursued here.

A Right to What?

It should be obvious that no claim of the form, "persons have a right to X" can be addressed without determining what kind of entity X is. Unless one is clear about what type of good health care is, resulting appraisals of its value and proper apportionment are hobbled. It will be suggested below that arguments for the provision of national health care pay insufficient attention to the changed and changing nature of health care. Three considerations are preliminary to that argument.

First, "health care" denotes a broad, ill-defined genus. Curative and preventive measures differ widely in their urgency; physicians vaccinate the young but also shore up sagging breasts and buttocks. In addition to activities centered around cure or prevention, health personnel carry out a large number of functions that bear little relation to combating disease. In their "caring" role they reassure the healthy,

---

Health Care: Issues and Directions for the Future," *American Journal of Orthopsychiatry* 42 (1972): 119-136; David Whipple, "Health Care as a Right: Its Economic Implications," *Inquiry* 11 (1974): 65-68; Bernard Williams, "The Idea of Equality," in *Problems of the Self* (London: Cambridge University Press, 1973), pp. 230-249.

2. For example, see Robert Nozick, *Anarchy, State and Utopia* (New York: Basic Books, 1974), pp. 232-235; Robert M. Sade, "Medical Care as a Right: A Refutation," *New England Journal of Medicine* 285 (2 December 1971): 1288-1292; Thomas Szasz "The Right to Health," *Georgetown Law Journal* 57 (1969): 734-751.

lend a sympathetic ear to complaints they cannot alleviate, provide counseling that, in a previous age, would have been sought from the clergy, lead the dying out of this life, and comfort the bereaved. Moreover, the range of services continues to expand as the medical profession is called upon to carry out tasks formerly performed by other social institutions. Nursing home expenditures multiply more rapidly than any other area within the system of health care delivery. The essentially custodial services they provide were, in the recent past, largely performed by the extended family. Their medicalization proceeds, not from any inner logic, but from extraneous social pressure.[3]

This diversity among health-care goods is one factor suggesting the desirability of shifting from broad discussions of health care as a right to the examination of *particular services* and their optimal distribution.

Second, no matter how wealthy a society is, its resources are never equal to the total number of demands placed upon them. Scarcity of goods relative to the possible ways in which they might usefully be employed is the basic postulate of economic science. The opportunity cost of using a resource in one way is the next best use forgone.[1] Only if a resource has no alternative uses is it free of cost.

Health care services compete amongst themselves for resources. They also compete with goods quite unrelated to health care. The very success with which they do so is, ironically, a major component of the "crisis" in health care. In 1955, health care expenditures accounted for 4.5 percent of the gross national product of the United States. By 1976 GNP had increased more than 300 percent, yet health care now took 8.7 percent of that much larger pie.[5] Every dollar spent represents other human wants that go unfulfilled. Again, reference to general health care rights seems less helpful than a close scrutiny of individual component services.

Third, is it within the power of governments to provide full and equal access to health care? If not, then there exists no right to it.

3. Victor Fuchs, "Economics, Health and Post-Industrial Society," *Milbank Memorial Fund Quarterly* 57 (1979): 165-167.

4. See James M. Buchanan, *Cost and Choice* (Chicago: Markham Publishing Company, 1969).

5. U. S. Department of Health Education and Welfare, *Health, United States, 1978* (Washington, D.C.: Government Printing Office), p. 380.

Every right must be a right against some specifiable person or group
of persons and is a claim for the performance (or omission) of actions
which can be brought about (or avoided) by the party in question. For
example, in underdeveloped countries beset by a paucity of physicians
and supporting medical facilities, there can be no right against the
state for extensive health-care services. Wealthy nations are blessed
with ample medical resources and possess the authority to marshal
them for socially desirable goals. Affluence, however, does not eliminate, but instead transforms, the burden of providing full and equal
health services.

The first large-scale campaign for universal health insurance in the
United States dates back to World War I.[6] At that time Americans
were far less wealthy than they are now. Paradoxically, however, they
were better equipped to provide genuinely full and equal access to
health services. Medicine's power to intervene effectively in crises was
then extremely limited. Patients recovered in short order or died, in
either case removing themselves from the need for ongoing attention.
Chronic diseases, especially those associated with aging, were predom-
inantly dealt with outside of medical contexts. In consequence, little
extra benefit could be accorded the richest patients beyond what was
available to those of more modest means.

In the last quarter of the twentieth century, however, there exist
numerous high technology procedures that can be provided to only a
fraction of those who could benefit from them. Computerized axial
tomography, organ transplants, and coronary arteriograms are but
three conspicuous therapeutic measures whose use is limited by
financial or biological factors.[7] It is incumbent upon those who
demand that medical care of the highest quality be universally provided as a matter of right to explain how this can be done. And if it
cannot, which would they dispense with: equity or the lives that could

6. Daniel S. Hirschfield, *The Lost Reform* (Cambridge: Harvard University
Press, 1970).

7. See, respectively Stuart Shapiro and Stanley Wyman, "CAT Fever," *New
England Journal of Medicine* 294 (22 April 1976): 954-956; Nicholas Rescher.
"The Allocation of Exotic Medical Lifesaving Therapy," *Ethics* 79 (1969): 173-
174; Howard H. Hiatt, "Protecting the Medical Commons: Who is Responsible?"
New England Journal of Medicine 293 (31 July 1975): 237.

be saved by selective use of expensive technology? (I shall return later to this dilemma.)

The preceding remarks suggest that there is a wide gulf between medical care being an important human *interest* or *need* and its being a *right*. Interests admit of a wide range of degree and can be freely traded off, one for another. Needs are interests that possess a high degree of urgency, but carry no explicit entitlement to the goods or services of other people. Rights, though, are demands that others *must* comply with; where compliance is impossible or unwarranted, no right exists.

The Welfare Case for a National Health Program

Even if health care in all its dimensions cannot, strictly speaking, be made out to be a human right, proponents of a national health program can argue that it is a good that ought to be provided to all irrespective of the ability to pay. Economic impoverishment would no longer follow in the wake of major illness. Government would be able to address directly the problem of ever rising costs instead of trying to influence at arm's length the fragmented health care industry. Finally, a more rational allocation of scarce medical resources to those who are most in need of them would be achieved. The de facto rationing of services by the market would be replaced by explicit consideration of how most equitably to optimize benefits for a given level of expenditure.

Major medical treatments *are* enormously expensive; for many persons the expense occasioned by an illness is its most persistent burden. We are all roughly equal in our vulnerability to debilitating disease or accident. Therefore, everyone would receive benefit from a national health plan that removed the threat of impoverishment as a consequence of medical disability. But this end can be achieved equally well by less sweeping measures. The risk of large economic loss can easily be guarded against by insurance. Its characteristic function is to protect against infrequent, unpredictable events which, when aggregated over a large population, are statistically regular.

Medical insurance is readily available in a variety of forms from private insurance companies. Like fire, automobile, and life insurance, it offers a means for persons to pool economic risks that are too great to hazard on an individual basis. Health maintenance organizations (HMOs) represent another and growing means by which prepayment allows individuals to spread risks. (In addition, HMOs offer service providers added inducement to economize on hospital stays and questionable surgical intervention, thus moderating overall medical expenditures.)[8] The special problems of the poor can be met by cash grants or by health-care vouchers exchangeable for prepaid services. Given the availability of these sharply focused means for dealing with unpredictable expense, the threat of major economic loss cannot provide a sound justification for a national health program.

Ever-rising total health care expenditure creates a different dilemma, one that is also far more unyielding. As long as the demand for medical services (especially those embracing high technology) keeps growing, continuous cost increases largely represent an efficient response to consumers' preferences.[9] Of course, these preferences can be questioned. Critics of prevailing practices have frequently argued that a more rational allocation of resources would redirect funds away from costly acute intervention procedures to preventive medicine and health education. However, even if this shift in emphasis could be carried out, benefits might prove to be less than anticipated. Annual physical checkups have long been advocated as worthwhile prophylaxis. Although they clearly impose substantial burdens on health care delivery systems, there is little evidence demonstrating significant health gains.[10] Routine mammography to detect breast cancer is now believed to cause more cancer than it uncovers.[11]

Education to alter unhealthy lifestyles would undoubtedly have a momentous positive impact—if we know how to provide it. Wide dis-

8. An important recent study is Jon B. Christianson and Walter McClure, "Competition in the Delivery of Health Care," *New England Journal of Medicine* 301 (11 October 1979): 812-818.

9. See Edmond D. Pellegrino, "Medical Economics and Morality: The Conflict of Canons," *Hospital Progress* 59 (August 1978): 50-55.

10. Richard Spark, "The Case Against Regular Physicals," *New York Times Magazine*, 25 July 1976, pp. 10 ff.

11. John Bailar, "Mammography—A Time for Caution," *Journal of the American Medical Association* 237 (7 March 1977): 997-998; Samuel Thier, "Breast Cancer Screening: A View from Outside the Controversy," *New England Journal of Medicine* 297 (10 November 1977): 1063-1065.

semination of the relevant information may accomplish little: there is
probably not a smoker in the country unaware of cigarettes' dele-
terious effects or a motorcyclist uninformed about the dangers of rid-
ing helmetless. In a free society there are limits to how much good one
can do for another who is not very interested.

Governmental control typically features politically motivated decisions and cozy relationships between an industry and its regulators
that work against economic efficiency.[12] In addition, there are good
reasons to believe that a national health program would be even *more
susceptible* to escalating costs than most federal ventures. First, to be
workable it would need the support of health professionals. It is therefore unlikely that they will be pressured to accept lower fees in order
to realize monetary savings. Witness the boon to physicians' incomes
provided by Medicare. Second, few citizens clamor for the purchase
of another battleship, and even highly subsidized train fares move few
people out of automobiles and airplanes. But health care is a commodity that most people desire. To lower or eliminate out-of-pocket
expenses for it will predictably increase demand and thus further burden the public purse. Costs may be shared more evenly, but
they will not be small.

The only way a nationalized program can realistically hope to keep
costs in line is to enforce strict schedules of permissible treatments for
all illnesses. These would be established on the basis of empirical
studies detailing cost-effectiveness—assuming that political pressures
to act otherwise are avoided. Therapeutic measures failing to come
up to the stipulated benefit-per-dollar level would simply be disallowed.
In effect, the goal of moderating overall costs would be subsumed
under that of equitable rationing. So, if the case for a national health
program can be made at all, it is on the grounds of enforcing the equal
provision of health services based solely on need.

Equality and Health Care

The case for equality in the delivery of health-care services may be
presented as simply one specification of the general brief for economic
equality. But then it is subject to all the standard criticisms that beset

12. Richard Posner, "Regulatory Aspects of National Health Insurance
Plans," *University of Chicago Law Review* 39 (Fall 1971): pp. 1-29.

rigid egalitarianism. If equality of condition is to be enforced, the liberty to pursue projects that generate differential rewards must be restricted. Substitutes must be found for the motivating force provided by the desire to better one's estate and the fear of seeing it diminished. The intuition that some merit more than others in return for greater effort or services rendered must be set aside. In short, the single-minded pursuit of equality is exceedingly costly in terms of other values surrendered, other goods forgone.

An alternative defense focuses on the special nature of health. The value of experiencing grand opera, vintage Chablis, a Yankee-Red Sox doubleheader or a trek up a mountain will vary greatly from individual to individual. Differences in talents and preferences will render ludicrous any program intent on providing these goods in equal measure to the entire populace. It is clearly preferable to allow individuals to pursue them as they will. But health is different. Whatever else one wants, good health is not only wanted but needed. Failure in securing it jeopardizes all other attainments. Moreover, its absence is rarely an indication of culpability; it is bad luck. Coordinated activity of men in civil society cannot abolish luck but it can ameliorate the stark randomness of its effects. The case for treating health care as a public good, subsidized by the common treasure, is that to do so is the most effective way we have of counteracting the vagaries of nature and providing each person with the preconditions for living a satisfying life.

Classical liberalism's "night watchman" state is devoted to the maximization of liberty, not equality. Yet it is committed to the equal protection of individuals against aggression. It singles out defense as a special good, one to be provided equally to all irrespective of the ability to pay for it.[13] Both aggression and disease are threats to the security of the individual, and one need not have incurred any prior culpability to be vulnerable. Just as civil society and the goods it provides human beings cannot endure in the face of unchecked aggression, the pursuit of individually meaningful projects presupposes minimal standards of physiological functioning. The institution of civil society neutralizes natural advantages possessed in a state of nature by the strong over the weak; similarly, public provision of

13. See the discussion in Robert Nozick, *Anarchy, State and Utopia*, pp. 26-28.

medical services would mitigate the advantages possessed by the healthy over the sick. Finally, both security from aggression and health are universally regarded as desirable. In securing them, the state is providing its citizens what they *need* and (except for aberrant cases) what they *want*. Thus, no class within society is being favored over any other. An outcome desired by all, and tending to be of equal benefit to all, is a prime candidate on grounds of justice and welfare for public advancement.

The analogy is not perfect. National defense is a public good in the economists' sense of being difficult or impossible to provide to one segment of the community without being extended willy-nilly to all others. Thus, if it were purchased in market transactions by independently acting persons, the existence of free riders would tend to lead to underconsumption relative to the optimum quantity of protection desired. With the exception of some public health measures such as immunization against contagious diseases and the removal of toxic substances from the environment, health services are generally not marked by externalities generating free riders.[14]

A more serious objection to the analogy is that states, of necessity, possess a monopoly on the exercise of coercive force.[15] Being the sole possessors of a right to exercise coercion, governments are obliged to undertake the functions of protection, apprehension, and punishment that citizens are prohibited from carrying out on an individual basis. There exists no similar necessity that states monopolize the provision of health services. Health may indeed be a primary human good, but whether it is distributed centrally or by independent contractors is irrelevant to the continued existence of a political order. That is not to deny that states have obligations to their citizenry respecting health care delivery. A state acts unjustly if it forbids crucial health services to some or all persons or if it promotes economic inequalities that deprive disadvantaged social classes of adequate medical care. It should be noted though that unjust health policies may appear either in states with comprehensive national health care or those without

14. James F. Blumstein and Michael Zubkoff, "Perspectives on Government Policy in the Health Sector," *Milbank Memorial Fund Quarterly* 51 (1973): 395-431.

15. For this characterization of the state see Max Weber, *Theory of Social and Economic Organization* (New York: Free Press, 1947), p. 156.

it. In either, services may be discriminatorily distributed, subverted for political ends, irrationally regulated, or irresponsive to consumer demand. The desirability of national health care cannot be deduced from a pure philosophical theory of justice; rather, its desirability hinges on whether, in the actual world, it promises to promote a fair and efficient allocation of resources.

The Changing Nature of Health Care

The enormous successes of medicine in the twentieth century have altered its face beyond recognition. Gone is the physician who, in his little black bag, carried almost all the essentials of his craft. Technology has dramatically enhanced medicine's power to extend lives, in some cases lives of a greatly diminished quality from that which we take to be optimally livable. Mortality and morbidity remain the chief antagonists of medical practitioners. Battle lines, however, have become blurred as success in warding off death actually increases the prevalence of certain pathological states. Dr. Ernest M. Gruenberg notes that

> In fact, as the result of advances in medical care we are seeing a rising prevalence of certain chronic conditions which previously led to early terminal infections, but whose victims now suffer from them for a longer period. The goal of medical research is to diminish disease and enrich life, but it produces tools which prolong diseased, diminished lives and so increase the proportion of people who have a disabling or chronic disease. . . . These increasingly common chronic conditions represent the failures of success. Their growing prevalence and longer duration are a product of progress in health technology.[16]

Among the conditions cited by Dr. Gruenberg are mongolism, senile brain damage, and spina bifida. Survival rates for those afflicted have increased dramatically, but little or no progress has been made in either preventing their occurrence or in restoring a semblance of normal functioning. The well-publicized (and anticlimactic) case of Karen Ann Quinlan brought home to many for the first time the fact

16. "The Failures of Success," *Milbank Memorial Fund Quarterly* 55 (1977): 5.

that medicine's ability to prolong life indefinitely may be not only costly but embarrassing. In restrospect, the 1930s and 1940s take on the
aspect of a golden age of curative medicine. Victories over disease
made possible by "miracle drugs" went hand in hand with victories
over death, and the benefits of medical intervention appeared incon-
testable and unalloyed. Since then not only have major advances been
harder to come by, but they are also marked by greater moral
ambiguity. That the application of lifesaving technology is always and
everywhere an indication of progress can no longer be safely assumed.

When is a therapeutic procedure proven to be a useful member
of the medical repertoire? Randomized controlled trials can demonstrate statistically whether a procedure has some effect. They cannot,
however, establish that results achieved are indeed benefits or that
they justify the costs incurred. These latter questions will be confronted in practice, even if by attempted abdications of responsibility.
What remains to be determined is who will pronounce on them: a
centralized governmental agency promulgating a unified national
health policy or millions of health service providers and consumers
acting independently?

Collective vs. Private Choice: Some Examples

A foretaste of the difficulties that would regularly confront a nationalized health program is provided by the debate over Medicaid
funded abortion.[17] Each year the nation is treated to a ritualized con-
gressional confrontation that changes no minds, produces no consensus, yet paralyzes essential legislative operations throughout its
duration. Few can believe that this public fanning of already polarized
attitudes is worthwhile; yet there seems to be no way to avoid it so long
as the provision of specific medical services to the poor remains an
item for legislative decision. The right of women to procure abortions
may have been conclusively established by judicial action, but a
democracy must also recognize the right of individual citizens to
participate in processes determining how their tax monies will be
spent. Either the public treasure will release funds to pay for abortion
or it will not; room for compromise is narrowly constricted.

17. See Thomas Schelling, "Standards for Adequate Minimum Personal Health
Services," *Milbank Memorial Fund Quarterly* 57 (1979): 212-233.

Entirely removing abortion related issues from the public agenda may be neither feasible nor desirable. But this especially futile contest is the direct product of choosing to meet the health needs of the poor through a centrally funded and regulated program. If Medicaid and related welfare measures were replaced by a negative income tax or some other device guaranteeing all persons a minimally adequate income, recipients would be free to purchase those goods and services of greatest personal urgency. Poor persons, if they so chose, could avail themselves of abortions on the same basis as other members of the population. A less sweeping alteration of current welfare programs would be to provide health care vouchers.[18] In either case, we would be spared a situation in which others decide for the poor what specific services they can or cannot have. Perhaps these proposed alternatives are defective on other grounds, but they do point up the advantages of leaving medical questions that touch on basic values up to individual discretion.

By means of amniocentesis, dozens of hereditary fetal traits can presently be detected. They range from its sex to the presence of debilitating diseases such as Tay-Sachs or mongolism. Occasionally the procedure is useful for diagnosing a condition that can be treated in utero, but it is also employed to procure information on which the decision whether or not to abort will be based. Will a national health program routinely provide amniocentesis when abortion is intended if results are negative? Or will it attempt somehow to keep to a middle course, allowing procedures leading to the abortion of severely in-

18. Vouchers are an intriguing device for coupling the attainment of social purposes with protection of personal autonomy. In addition, they are flexible: a restrictive voucher plan will resemble a centralized program while less restrictive ones are more like cash-grant schemes. In which direction should a health-care voucher plan lean? The question is thorny, but, on balance, a minimum of restrictions seems desirable because it allows for (1) respect for personal autonomy; (2) the (admittedly defeasible) conviction that individuals are better judges of their health-care preferences and needs than are boards of central planners; (3) competition, more needed by the health industry than enforced uniformity; (4) minimization of political wrangling over the inclusion of particular services such as abortion.

Against these must be weighed the paternalistic concern that individuals will misallocate their vouchers. Much work remains to be done in the foundations of voucher theory. Moral philosophers ought to be involved in this inquiry; the issues are too involved to be left exclusively to the economists.

capacitated fetuses but not, say, those of the parentally disfavored
sex? Alternatively, a cost-conscious program could require as a condition of coverage that women at risk undergo amniocentesis and abortion when a live birth will entail huge medical costs. These hypothetical policies are not of equal likelihood, but any one of them would
engender pitched battles whose outcome would certainly leave large
sections of the population dissatisfied. Pollyannas may expect the
passage of time to ease these problems. Just the reverse will be the
case; as techniques of genetic screening and engineering become more
sophisticated, moral quandries will ineluctably multiply. Sometimes
polarization is the inescapable consequence of forging a national
policy, but in this case divisiveness can be minimized by leaving decisions in the hands of private citizens.

The other end of human existence has also been profoundly affected
by advances in medical capabilities. The hospital has replaced the
home as the usual place to die, and it is increasingly the case that the
exact time of death is a matter for choice. Biological function can be
preserved in so attenuated a state that physicians have been forced
to move toward a redefinition of "death" in order to avoid the ghoulish
indefinite preservation of living corpses.[19] But most ethical dilemmas
surrounding death and dying are untouched by semantic legerdemain.
Unless one supposes that each advance in the power to sustain life
creates a corresponding imperative for its universal employment—and
also creates the funds to pay for them—there is no simple answer to
the question of when to extend life and when to terminate it. Here I
shall sidestep substantive matters to raise instead a procedural issue:
to what extent is it desirable that government intrude upon deliberations at the edge of life?

It is unrealistic to deny that the state does have some legitimate
interests. Inevitably it must confront practices that raise the specter
of homicide. The law must also establish standards concerning informed consent and the contractual obligations obtaining between
patient and physician. But beyond staking out legal terrain within
which concerned parties can take their bearings, government may

19. Ad Hoc Committee of the Harvard Medical School to Examine the Definition of Brain Death, "A Definition of Irreversible Coma," *Journal of the American Medical Association* 205 (5 August 1968): 337-340.

move in either of two opposed directions: it can issue detailed regulations pertaining to the application of lifesaving technology or, within broad guidelines, it can return decision-making prerogatives to individual patients, their families and physicians. For two major reasons, the latter course is to be preferred whenever possible.

First, individual discretion promotes autonomy. Persons differ in their judgments concerning the conditions under which life is no longer worth living. They will also vary in their willingness to forgo other possible satisfactions for the sake of securing incremental health gains. A liberal society is one that values the ability of individuals to direct their own lives. One signficant way in which this value can be pursued is to allow people to determine for themselves what course their medical treatments will take. A recent expression of this policy is the granting of legal status to "living wills," documents that spell out conditions under which the signator desires that heroic medical procedures be terminated. The gradual development of hospice programs also provides enhanced opportunities for terminally ill patients to take charge of their own destinies. Instead of being shunted aside as medicine's embarrassing failure, the hospice patient is encouraged to accept the fact of his upcoming death and to influence the conditions under which he will depart from life. As technology continually enlarges the scope for intervention into the process of dying, further methods will be required to ensure that the party most directly affected is able to play a significant role.

Second, an active governmental role in mandating standards for care poses the same danger of political disruption that has already been experienced in the case of publicly funded abortion. All citizens have a fundamental stake in how they and their loved ones will die. Decisions in this sphere do not come easily under the best of circumstances. But burdens will be exacerbated if matters of personal decision are transformed into public policy questions. Regulation is, in essence, inflexible. If national standards are to be formulated that adjudicate among basic and deeply felt values, diverse groups will want to see their own attitudes enshrined in law. A zero-sum game will develop in which one side's gain is another's loss, and so each will attempt to use the political machinery for its own ends.

If the state assumes full responsibility for the provision of health services, it will be unable to avoid dictating standards for the utilization of life sustaining services. Extraordinary means for staving off death are inordinately costly both in monetary terms and in demands placed upon highly trained personnel. If the ability of patients to pay is entirely removed as a factor influencing their use, there will be an increased call for their employment. To remain solvent, a national health program will have to contain some formula for determining when the cost of procuring and employing expensive technology are justified by realizable benefits. If such a formula is not to be subverted from within, little room for exceptions can be permitted. Whatever structure emerges is sure to leave many health professionals and consumers dissatisfied. They will be informed that their own personal discretion must give way to considerations of the public good—as defined by a distant bureaucracy.

It can be objected that constraints upon resources are inevitable regardless of the system by which health care is financed. Nationalization merely shifts the appraisal of costs and benefits from innumerable private hands to one central apparatus. Efficiency is thereby enhanced because policy will be consistently formulated by authorities possessing all the information needed to make rational decisions. Medical services will not be wastefully showered on patients simply because they are prepared to pay for them, nor will they be denied to persons of modest means. As a welcome fringe benefit, patients, their families, and physicians will be spared the necessity of making wrenching choices in cases where objectivity gives way to emotional pressure.

This response begs several crucial questions. Do health bureaucrats really possess more relevant information than individual practitioners and patients? Surely familiarity with a particular case must count for something. Health services are not provided to faceless pathological syndromes but to persons whose preferences and circumstances are endlessly varied and complexly interrelated. If responsiveness to individual differences is something worth prizing, it is morally obtuse to restrict attention only to data that can be quantified and processed by technocrats. A corollary surmise is that consistency in the dispensation of health resources may not be an unquestioned virtue; perhaps it is the compassionate willingness to accede to individual needs that instead ought to be consistently pursued. And is it a genuine welfare gain if individuals are denied the responsibility of making difficult choices in extremis? An affirmative answer reveals an implicit valuation of impotent contentment over psychically demanding self-direction. It is by no means clear that this represents an acceptable ranking.

Deciding when treatment shall cease involves ethical questions of considerable magnitude. A yet more vexing range of dilemmas surround triage: the selection of some for treatment when not all can be saved. If resources are indispensable to a group of persons at peril but too limited to accommodate all, to save one life is to sacrifice another. Our moral principles are severely strained by circumstances that require the balancing of one innocent life against another. Such choices, however, promise to intrude upon us increasingly.

Two classic examples of triage are the dangerously overloaded lifeboat and the harried medic patching up the wounded on a battlefield. Whatever is done, some salvageable lives will be forfeited. The dreadfulness of these choices, though, is somewhat softened by the urgency of a crisis: action must be immediate and there is little luxury for reflective deliberation. If called upon to justify his actions, an agent could plead that he was reacting instinctively to the needs of the moment.

Contemporary medical technology is responsible for triage situations of a rather different character. A mechanism is devised that is effective against some previously untreatable condition. Unfortunately, only a small percentage of those afflicted can receive treatment. Who shall be allowed to live? Here decision-makers are dealing with a series of events predictable well in advance. Not enmeshed in a precipitously developing crisis, they are privileged to assume the role of detached administrator. There is, however, a price to be paid for this relative ease: whatever standards are developed and employed are subject to close scrutiny. Those disfavored in the selection process are perfectly entitled to ask why. Persuasive answers will not be easily forthcoming.

It is useful to glance at the history of hemodialysis. By provisions of the Social Security Amendments of 1972 (Pl 92-603) the United

States Federal Government undertook to cover the costs of either dialysis or renal transplant for nearly all those who suffer from chronic kidney failure. Costs are extremely high—in the range of two billion dollars annually—but this massive infusion of funds has greatly increased the availability of dialysis machines and, even more importantly, the highly trained people needed to run kidney units.[20] Prior to 1972, however, dialysis treatment was available to only a minority of those persons who qualified for it on purely medical grounds. Centers that offered dialysis adopted diverse means for selecting among applicants who passed an initial screening. Some employed committees composed entirely of physicians while others used lay committees. Among the criteria utilized at various hospitals were first-come first-served, drawing lots, and evaluations of expected social worth.[21] The well-publicized chronic dialysis selection committee at the Seattle Artificial Kidney Center is reported to have considered whether applicants had been scout leaders, church members or Red Cross volunteers.[22] Two investigators of their procedures have aptly concluded that they rule out "creative nonconformists who rub the bourgeoisie the wrong way but who historically have contributed so much to the making of America. The Pacific Northwest is no place for a Henry David Thoreau with bad kidneys."[23]

I have not referred to this episode in order to pluck from it handy lessons concerning how triage decisions are best arrived at. I believe

20. See Richard Rettig, "Lessons Learned from the End-State Renal Disease Experience" in Richard Egdahl and Paul Gertman, eds., *Technology and the Quality of Health Care* (Germantown, MD: Aspen Systems Corporation, 1978), pp. 153-173; Eliot Marshal, "Rendezvous with a Machine," *New Republic* 176 (19 March 1977): 16-19.

21. Paul Ramsey, "Scarce Medical Resources," *Columbia Law Review* 69 (1969): 620-692; Jay Katz and Alexander Morgan Capron, *Catastrophic Diseases: Who Decides What?* (New York: Russell Sage Foundation, 1975), pp. 178-196.

22. See, especially, Shana Alexander, "They Decide Who Lives, Who Dies: Medical Miracle Puts a Moral Burden on a Small Committee," *Life* 53 (9 November 1962): 102 ff; Paul Ramsey, "Scarce Medical Resources," p. 659; Renee Fox and Judith Swazey, *The Courage to Fail* (Chicago: University of Chicago Press, 1974), pp. 240-279.

23. David Sanders and Jessee Dukeminier, Jr., "Medical Advance and Legal Lag: Hemodialysis and Kidney Transplantation," *UCLA Law Review* 15 (1968): 378.

that there are none. If the dialysis experience is instructive, it is in showing that we possess neither reliable intuitive nor theoretical grounds for making a choice of life against life. Because each human life is owed maximum respect, differential treatment based on precarious judgments of social worth is odious. But to consign individuals to life or death because of the results of a lottery allows impersonal forces to adjudicate in the most deeply personal of crises. Both procedures are more stopgaps than solutions—assuming that it is even possible to speak of a "solution" in such cases.[21] However, I want to address a further question: should triage decisions be left to numerous private groups acting independently, or should responsibility be assumed by a national health care delivery board?

The latter would, I believe, be a profoundly unsatisfactory state of affairs. The least of its drawbacks is that treatment decisions would be thrust into the arena of public choice where diverse groups would lobby intensively for special consideration. It requires little imagination to foresee the young, those with dependents, military veterans, persons holding responsible positions, and others all claiming to merit a preferred status. A policy of random selection might appease these contending forces, but it also might appear to each of them as unjustly slighting legitimate merit. The trouble arises precisely because no process of choice presents itself as clearly superior; whichever method is imposed will be open to objections rendering it unstable.

Consider a further complication: wealthy individuals may not be content to leave their survival to the vagaries of a national health care system. Suppose they choose to go outside of the system to procure lifesaving technology; how will authorities respond? If the rich are allowed carte blanche, the egalitarianism of national health care is compromised in a context where the stakes are no less than life and death. If outside access is forbidden by law, the situation is even more

24. References previously cited concerning the history of dialysis in the United States all deal at greater or lesser length with the ethical bases of triage. For theoretical discussions of this issue displaying significantly varied approaches, see James F. Childress, "Who Shall Live When Not All Can Live?" *Soundings* 53 (1970): 339-355; Nicholas Rescher, "The Allocation of Exotic Medical Lifesaving Therapy," and Robert Young, "Some Criteria for Making Decisions Concerning the Distribution of Scarce Medical Resources," both in *Theory and Decision* 6 (1975): 439-455.

anomalous. Persons who are entitled to spend their money for utterly frivolous purposes will be precluded from using it to remain alive.[25] No compensating gain for the poor would be realized—unless a surrender to envy is counted as a gain.

When triage decisions are made by dozens of independent private organizations, rejection is a bitter blow. But it is neither as final nor so laden with ominous overtones as rejection by a governmental board. If a candidate for treatment regards one hospital's selection criteria as unfair he can apply elsewhere. Or, if turned down at one, he may be able to succeed at another.

Rulings promulgated in the name of a national health monopoly are doubly definitive. They carry not only *finality* but also *authority*. Decisions exercised by a handful of administrators at a private hospital may reflect nothing beyond their own idiosyncratic values; national health care, however, serves the entire citizenry and is responsible to it. Triage is never unproblematic, but on what basis could a creature of the state adopt *any* principle of selection? Whoever is excluded can justifiably complain that he is thereby being disadvantaged by the very institution whose special duty is to extend equal protection to all persons. The essential point is not that government will do a poorer job of allocating lifesaving technology than would non-governmental units—although, given the nature of the political pressures to which it is subject, it very well might—but that *this is a singularly inappropriate area for any governmental choice*, no matter how conscientiously it is made. Neutrality among all citizens is a political ideal that is easily subverted and, once breached, difficult to restore. I suggest that this ideal is well worth preserving, and that to establish a precedent of forcing the state to determine that some named individuals shall live and others die is to do that ideal possibly irreparable damage. When such decisions have to be made, it is far better that they be carried out by non-public boards not constrained by obligations of equal protection to an entire citizenry. Flexibility is enhanced, and the implications of unsavory choices are localized.

One objection to this argument is that government can and should avoid the necessity of triage by providing resources sufficient to ac-

25. This problem is raised by Charles Fried, "Equality and Rights in Medical Care," *Hastings Center Report* 6 (1976) p. 31.

commodate all patients. Indeed, precisely this intent motivated the passage of the 1972 legislation providing dialysis treatment to all end-stage renal disease sufferers in need of it. Could not a well-funded national health-care program act similarly in all other cases?

The answer is no. There are some shortages that not even unlimited finances can eliminate. The number of persons who can be benefited by organ transplants already exceeds the available supply. As further advances in immunosuppression and surgical technique are realized, the disparity will grow. Transplantable hearts cannot be produced by governmental edict. Further, there is always a gap between the time a procedure is experimentally introduced and its widespread implementation.

In the real world, finances are not unlimited. Money used to counter one life-threatening syndrome is unavailable for others. For example, the huge infusion of Medicare funds for kidney disease sufferers could have been devoted to the comparably expensive treatment of hemophiliacs. That it was not may be due only to the greater muscle of the kidney disease lobby. Even if sufficient funds to eliminate all triage situations could be raised, it does not follow that to do so is advisable. A commitment to treat every salvageable patient will shortchange other legitimate health goals as well as competing goods in other spheres. An ironic result of nationalized health care might be that to avoid the undoubted evil of governmental triage, grotesque misallocations of resources will ensue. Is it really desirable that education, housing and general economic advancement be penalized so that a 110-year-old patient can receive his third kidney transplant and second artificial heart?

National Health Care and Non-Standard Options

The terms with which a debate is pursued can become frozen while the underlying real dimensions continue to change. This has been the fate of the case for national health care. Its desirability cannot be assessed in a vacuum; as the nature of the commodity health care evolves so too do reasons for and against its provision by the state. The most revolutionary development in medical practice since national health care was initially broached is the increasing prominence of *non-standard options*. By "non-standard option" I mean a medical service possessing the following three features: (1) Each occasion on which it is delivered entails great expense; (2) It has little effect on mortality or morbidity configurations for the population as a whole; (3) Individuals who receive the service are substantially benefited or perceive themselves to be substantially benefited.

Proliferation of non-standard options bedevils egalitarianism in health care delivery. A system that undertook to fulfill all requests on the basis of demonstrated need at no charge to recipients would soon be bankrupt. If non-standard options were excluded from the system but could be secured privately, major inequalities in health-care delivery would thereby be reintroduced. Finally, if non-standard options that cannot be offered to all are forbidden to all, government is placed in the uncomfortable position of abridging the liberty of citizens to preserve health and life.

Health-care delivery has often been cited as an area in which the case for equality is especially convincing, even self-evident. In an important paper, Bernard Williams has maintained that, "leaving aside preventive medicine, the proper ground of distribution of medical care is ill health: this is a necessary truth."[26] I have argued that it is not a necessary truth but rather a seductive falsehood based on an obsolete model of medical care. It does indeed seem intolerable that anyone should die or continue to suffer from disease when, for a relatively small expenditure, his plight can be alleviated. Even on coldly economic grounds, it is irrational not to invest a sum that will be returned many times over in a life of increased productivity. But non-standard options do not fit this model. Their opportunity costs are extremely high, they rarely provide restoration to full health, and the need for them continually outstrips the available supply.[27]

26. "The Idea of Equality," p. 240.

27. Governmentally provided Catastrophic Health Insurance (coverage for medical expenses above a stipulated minimum) has often been urged as a compromise between a comprehensive national health program and the status quo. Several objections to this policy have been frequently rehearsed: incentives are increased for the use of costly hospital service in place of less costly alternatives; once the floor expenditure has been reached, patients and physicians will have little incentive to minimize further therapy; major medical health insurance is readily available from the private sector. But the foregoing discussion suggests an even more far-reaching objection: non-standard options would, of course, all qualify financially as catastrophic expenses. It would be

Suggestions for a Medical Marketplace

I have been arguing that national health care is an idea whose time has come—and gone. That should not be interpreted as a brief for the status quo. Ongoing expansion of the medical role argues against imposing uniformity in the delivery of health services. It is not enough, however, to reject national health care; positive steps should be taken to enable consumers to choose for themselves the goods and services they most want. This requires a genuine marketplace: a sector in which alternative products are offered and where those who receive a good are the ones who pay for it. I conclude with five brief suggestions concerning how diversity and consumer sovereignty can be enhanced.

First, there are better and worse means by which society can respond to the health needs of the poor. Routing all medical care through a monolithic national health service has already been amply criticized. Somewhat preferable would be the provision of a suitably defined "minimum decent standard" of health care. One drawback of this proposal is that not all will agree on what counts as minimally decent. The acrimonious debate over Medicaid funded abortion is a case in point. Also, the poor will still be precluded from acting on their own preferences. Therefore, I suggest instead a cash grant or voucher program enabling the poor to purchase their own medical services on a prepaid basis. How generous this program should be is a crucial question that cannot be explored in this paper.

Second, influential health-care spokespersons should avoid making extravagant claims heralding the accomplishments of highpowered medicine. Such statements lead to unrealistic expectations on the part of consumers and consequent pressure upon the health care system to deliver more than it is capable of providing. Newly developed technology provides genuine health gains, but its effect on mortality and morbidity are inconsequential compared to the dramatic gains realized between the 1930s and 1950s. Predictions are hazardous, but we very probably have reached a point of drastically diminishing returns on the health care dollar. Pessimism concerning future health gains need not follow: health care is not the same as health. There are a great

---

ironic indeed if universal catastrophic coverage were enacted just as the progress of medical technology renders its provision unattainable.

number of steps individuals can take to live longer and healthier lives: avoid smoking, eat breakfasts, get and stay married (especially significant for males), sleep at least seven hours each night, consume alcohol in moderation. These "life-style" patterns are free of cost, undeliverable by professionals, but wonderfully responsive to individual choice. Because what individuals can do for themselves far exceeds what can be done for them, we ought to begin to emphasize the former.[28]

Third, there is need to expand the variety of health-insurance policies and other prepaid packages. Not everyone needs or desires the same level of coverage. I see no reason to suppose that consumers are generally unable to choose rationally how much of their resources to devote to health goods. Nor is there any evidence that welfare gains are realized if central planning boards are vested with the responsibility for such choices. Some persons are very sensitive to increased probabilities of an extended life span; they ought to have the opportunity to purchase expensive policies that include coverage for a wide range of non-standard options. Those who place a premium on present consumption should be free to devote only a minimal amount of income to health care coverage. Both will thus be able to maximize expected utility while assuming responsibility for their own choices. A not incidental benefit is that triage dilemmas will be minimized; or rather, *individuals will be making such decisions for themselves* through genuine market arrangements. The prospective demand for some item of expensive lifesaving technology will tend to create its own supply.

Fourth, consumers of medical services will never reclaim control of their health care programs until what Charles Fried characterizes as "a guild system as tight and self-protective as any we know" is broken.[29] Physicians make virtually all medical decisions and are loath to relinquish any of this power either to public agencies or to consumers. Even the choice of a primary care physician is usually made blind because organized medicine has traditionally execrated advertising or any other means which would afford consumers the basis for

28. See the discussion in Chapter 2 of Victor Fuchs *Who Shall Live?* pp. 30-55.

29. Fried, "Equality and Rights in Medical Care," p. 33.

making a cost-conscious selection. Physicians' domination of health-care delivery is made possible by a legal structure that grants them unparalleled powers to control entry into the profession, set fees, and regulate their own practice. The results are remarkably high incomes and an almost total immunity from normal market forces. Numerous steps could be undertaken to transform this cartel into competitive purveyors of service to an informed clientele: eliminating all bans on advertising, easing the formation of HMOs and other alternatives to fee-for-service medicine, eliminating or drastically abridging entry restricting requirements, allowing patients and pharmacists more say in the selection of prescription drugs, and enabling other health professionals to provide services that do not require a physician's expertise.

Fifth, what ought to be done to hold down the nation's spiraling medical bill? Nothing. To be more precise, external bureaucratic regulation is the wrong prescription for the ills of our health care delivery system. If, as I have suggested above, consumers are afforded the opportunity to make informed purchases in a genuine medical marketplace, they will be able to determine what percentage of their income is devoted to health care. Is 5% of GNP too little, 15% too much? I suggest that there is no a priori answer to these questions. Health care is one among many services persons can choose for themselves in whatever quantity they desire—if they are given the chance to do so.

I would like to thank Paul Menzel, John Troyer and the Editors of *Philosophy & Public Affairs* for numerous helpful suggestions.

KENNETH J. ARROW   Gifts and Exchanges[1]

Richard Titmuss is justly distinguished for his devotion to the welfare of society at large and particularly to those who have received the least of society's benefits. He has not rested content with the moral satisfaction of advocating the good but has immersed himself in the detailed factual analysis and speculative thinking needed if good intentions are to become good deeds. The gift he has made of his talents has now found an appropriate embodiment in his latest and much-noticed study, *The Gift Relationship: From Human Blood to Social Policy.*[2] The study focuses specifically on the workings of a particular supply system, that by which blood is made available for transfusions in the United States and in the United Kingdom, with some reference to other nations. But this close study is intended as something of a searchlight to illuminate a much broader landscape: the limits of economic analysis, the rival uses of exchange and gift as modes of allocation, the collective or communitarian possibilities in society as against the tendencies toward individuaiism. Most of the discussion takes place in the precise and objective language of empirical sociology: surveys and tables are presented, the limits of the data are stated with the utmost care, but every now and then the strength of Titmuss' convictions shines forth. Perhaps the flavor of the lessons

1. Presented at the Conference on Altruism and Economic Theory held by the Russell Sage Foundation, 3-4 May 1972 (prepared with the partial support of NSF Grant GS-28626X, Harvard University).
2. (London and New York, 1971.) All page references in the text are to *The Gift Relationship.*

he wants us to learn can best be suggested by a somewhat lengthy quotation of his final two paragraphs:

> From our study of the private market in blood in the United States, we have concluded that the commercialization of blood and donor relationships represses the expression of altruism, erodes the sense of community, lowers scientific standards, limits both personal and professional freedoms, sanctions the making of profits in hospitals and clinical laboratories, legalizes hostility between doctor and patient, subjects critical areas of medicine to laws of the marketplace, places immense social costs on those least able to bear them—the poor, the sick, and the inept—increases the danger of unethical behavior in various sectors of medical science and practice, and results in situations in which proportionately more and more blood is supplied by the poor, the unskilled, the unemployed, Negroes and other low-income groups, and categories of exploited human populations of high blood yielders. Redistribution in terms of blood and blood products from the poor to the rich appears to be one of the dominant effects of the American blood-banking systems.
>
> Moreover, on four testable non-ethical criteria the commercialized blood market is bad. In terms of economic efficiency it is highly wasteful of blood; shortages, chronic and acute, characterize the demand-and-supply position and make illusory the concept of equilibrium. It is administratively inefficient and results in more bureaucratization and much greater administrative, accounting, and computer overheads. In terms of price per unit of blood to the patient (or consumer), it is a system which is five to fifteen times more costly than voluntary systems in Britain. And, finally, in terms of quality, commercial markets are much more likely to distribute the contaminated blood; the risks for the patient of disease and death are substantially greater. Freedom from disability is inseparable from altruism.

The present essay is a series of reflections on the descriptive and prescriptive issues raised by Titmuss' evidence and assertions. It is obvious on the most superficial observation that the allocation of goods and services is not accomplished entirely by exchange, as standard economic models would hold. Clearly this is true for such impalpable

goods as respect, love, or status, but even when we confine ourselves
to goods whose allocation the economist believes himself capable of
analyzing with his tools, the donation of blood for transfusions is only
one example of a large class of unilateral transactions in which there
is no element of payment in any direct or ordinary sense of the term.
Formal philanthropy has always been a prominent element of all economic systems and has shown no signs of diminution. Long ago
Kropotkin pointed out the vast amount of informal and irregular
mutual help given in times of need.[3] Of course, the whole structure
of government expenditures is a departure from the system of mutual
exchange. It is true that it has its own logic of coercion, so that it is
not quite an example of pure altruism, but in a democratic society the
voting of expenditures for the benefit of others plainly constitutes an
institutionalization of giving. Nor are gifts solely in the form of
money. The contribution of personal services, services which may
well involve significant personal costs or which could command a
considerable market value, for voluntary cooperative efforts of one
kind or another remains a prominent feature of social life, even—or
perhaps especially—in the United States, a country that Titmuss holds
up as the very model of a society atomized by excessive reliance on
the dictates of the marketplace.

There is another and very important sense in which a more subtle
form of giving affects the allocation of economic resources. It can be
argued that the presence of what are in a slightly old-fashioned terminology called *virtues* in fact plays a significant role in the operation
of the economic system. Titmuss calls attention to the great value of
truthfulness on the part of blood donors; the most serious risk in
blood transfusion is the possible transmission of serum hepatitis from
donor to recipient. Since no adequate test has yet been devised for
the presence of hepatitis in the blood, its detection depends essentially
on the willingness of the donor to state correctly whether or not he is
suffering from that disease. This is a prototype of many other similar
situations in economic life. Many of us consider it possible that the
process of exchange requires or at least is greatly facilitated by the
presence of several of these virtues (not only truth, but also trust,

3. Petr A. Kropotkin, *Mutual Aid: A Factor of Evolution* (London, 1902),
chap. VIII.

loyalty, and justice in future dealings). Now virtue may not always be its own reward, but in any case it is not usually bought and paid for at market rates. In short, the supply of a commodity in many respects complementary to those usually thought of as economic goods is not itself accomplished in the marketplace but rather comes as an unrequited transfer.

Finally, there is a broader set of issues raised by Titmuss. The picture of a society run exclusively on the basis of exchange has long haunted sensitive observers, especially from the early days of the capitalist domination. The ideas of community and social cohesion are counterposed to a drastically reduced society in which individuals meet only as buyers and sellers of commodities. Of course, giving is not the only alternative to a system of pure exchange. Authority and hierarchy constitute one alternative system, rational bureaucracy with place determined by merit another; but certainly the role of free giving in producing a more humanitarian social order is worth considering.

The points raised above determine the organization of the rest of this discussion. I shall consider in turn the role of giving as an expression of individual volition, as a contribution to economic efficiency, and as a determinant of social cohesion.

One further remark. As Titmuss indicates very clearly, the giving of blood is giving not to specific individuals but to an anonymous recipient. The motives for such giving are regarded as more definitely altruistic than those for giving to individuals. In what follows the discussion is therefore confined to impersonal giving.

I shall take for granted in most cases that Titmuss' empirical analysis is correct and concentrate rather on setting it in other contexts, though some comment on the evidence is unavoidable. I shall conclude with a further, though still cursory, examination of the extent to which in fact the empirical evidence he advances proves or at least strongly supports his various theses.

I. THE INDIVIDUAL'S DESIRE TO GIVE

The starting point of Titmuss' analysis and reflections is the basic fact that in the United Kingdom the supplying of blood for transfusions is completely voluntary and unpaid, while in the United States there is a mixed system with both commercial and noncommercial blood banks and with payments of various kinds. According to Titmuss' estimates, based on admittedly unsatisfactory surveys, about one-third of the United States supply (including derivatives such as plasma, plasma fractions, and red blood cell concentrates) comes from paid blood donors. Nor are the rest considered to be truly voluntary; by Titmuss' standards a donor is considered to be voluntary only if the recipient is unknown to him and there are no social sanctions enforcing the donation. Thus only 9 percent of the United States donors are regarded as voluntary. About one-half give blood free of charge, but in most cases they are in effect replacing blood given to relatives.

These figures, needless to say, are subject to a wide margin of error (the categories above are not completely exhaustive; I omit a few minor ones for the sake of simplicity). In the United Kingdom there are, of course, no paid donors. However, Titmuss has not attempted to classify the British donors in a comparable way, though in fact he has better evidence (mainly the results of a questionnaire survey which he himself developed). It does turn out that in the case of 28 percent of the British donors either they or their families have received blood transfusions.

As might be supposed, the distribution of blood donations between paid and unpaid donors influences the distribution of blood-giving among socio-economic categories. A rough impression of the fragmentary United States data together with that for the United Kingdom suggests that unpaid donations are distributed among socio-economic classes more or less in proportion to the relative size of each class. Paid donors, on the contrary, are drawn almost exclusively from the lower-income categories, including the unemployed.[4]

Even in the United Kingdom the percentage of the eligible population that gives blood is actually very small, only 6 percent according to Titmuss' estimates. Titmuss does not comment on this fact. The picture of a broadly altruistic society seems somewhat blurred when

4. One curious piece of data is that in the United States blood donors are overwhelmingly male, even among unpaid groups, while in the United Kingdom the donors are distributed between the sexes in the same proportion as that of men to women in the general population. Titmuss does not remark on this, and I have no explanatory hypothesis.

we realize what a small fraction of the population is in fact functioning altruistically.

It may be inferred from Titmuss' presentation that the motives for giving blood can be divided into three types: a generalized desire to benefit others, a feeling of social obligation, and a response to personal social pressures, as in the case of donations to known recipients or responses to institutional blood drives. I suggest here a reformulation of the first two of these motives in the language of utility theory. I find three classes, which do not correspond precisely to those of Titmuss:

(1) The welfare of each individual will depend both on his own satisfaction and on the satisfactions obtained by others. We here have in mind a positive relation, one of altruism rather than envy.

(2) The welfare of each individual depends not only on the utilities of himself and others but also on his contributions to the utilities of others.

(3) Each individual is, in some ultimate sense, motivated by purely egoistic satisfaction derived from the goods accruing to him, but there is an implicit social contract such that each performs duties for the other in a way calculated to enhance the satisfaction of all.[5]

This classification is not exhaustive, or even exclusive.

In (1) and (2), one is to distinguish between two levels of utility: each individual may be regarded as deriving satisfaction from the goods he receives, but his overall aim is to maximize welfare, a function of the satisfactions of all; he derives a utility from seeing someone else's satisfaction increased. The second version differs from the first only in that welfare is derived not merely from an increase in someone else's satisfaction but from the fact that the individual himself has contributed to that satisfaction. The first hypothesis has been used occasionally by economists in trying to explain why people give to others or why they vote for redistribution of income. But it does not seem very appropriate for the case of giving blood, especially with anonymous recipients. The utilities of all others would have to enter the welfare function in a completely symmetrical fashion. It does appear necessary to supplement this motivation with the additional

5. I am indebted to Thomas Nagel for some illuminating comments on these points.

measure of satisfaction derived from the fact that I, rather than some-one else, have brought about the improvement in social welfare. Put another way, under the first hypothesis I would prefer that you rather than I give to a third individual, but in the second case I might well prefer to give myself, because I would have the satisfaction of per-sonal participation in social welfare.

The third possible hypothesis is, according to my understanding, in the spirit of Kant's categorical imperative or Rawls's theory of jus-tice. In real life, however, emphasis must be put on the implicit nature of the social contract. One might be thought of as giving blood in the vague expectation that one may need it later on. More generally, per-haps, one gives good things, such as blood, in exchange for a general-ized obligation on the part of fellow men to help in other circum-stances if needed. Some of the subtleties of the social contract theory are seen when the anonymous recipients in question are future gen-erations or indeed the sick and poor of the present generation. Actual behavior, as reflected in decisions of democratic governments, shows that individuals are in fact willing to sacrifice present satisfactions for future generations, as in the case of public investments, or even for others living in the present, as evidenced by willingness on the part of middle-class citizens to vote for county hospitals while they themselves in fact use voluntary hospitals. Similarly, in voting for edu-cational expenditures, there must be many advocates of greater expenditure who do not have children who will benefit. One can try to rationalize their behavior either in terms of one of the first two hypotheses or in terms of the social contract made with previous and future generations. How such a social contract is in fact carried out is another matter. There are, of course, cultural institutions which reinforce it; Kropotkin argued that there is a built-in evolutionary mechanism to this end, for altruism aids in the survival of the species, a thesis repeated more recently by Wynne-Edwards.[6]

Titmuss makes explicit a feeling held by many, I think, in his dis-cussion of what he calls in a chapter title "The Right to Give." Econo-mists typically take for granted that since the creation of a market increases the individual's area of choice it therefore leads to higher

6. V. C. Wynne-Edwards, *Animal Dispersion in Relation to Social Behavior* (New York, 1962).

benefits. Thus, if to a voluntary blood donor system we add the possibility of selling blood, we have only expanded the individual's range of alternatives. If he derives satisfaction from giving, it is argued, he can still give, and nothing has been done to impair that right. But this is emphatically not the view held by Titmuss. On the contrary, he states, "as this study has shown comparatively, private market systems in the United States and other countries . . . deprive men of their freedom to choose to give or not to give" (p. 239). Shortly thereafter he continues: "In a positive sense we believe that policy and processes should enable men to be free to choose to give to unnamed strangers. They should not be coerced or constrained by the market. In the interests of the freedom of all men, they should not, however, be free to sell their blood or decide on a specific destination of the gift. The choice between these claims—between different kinds of freedom—has to be a social policy decision; in other words, it is a moral and political decision for the society as a whole" (p. 242). I can find no support in the evidence for the existence of such a dilemma. Indeed, it is not easy to see what kind of evidence would be relevant. Presumably the best that could be done would be to show that the amount of blood given in the United States is less than it would be if commercial blood-giving were prohibited. In turn, this might be inferred from a comparison of the number of donors in the United States and in the United Kingdom. Titmuss nowhere makes any explicit comparison of this kind. I would in fact gather from his figures that the percentage of donors in the United States *is* lower than that in the United Kingdom, but since the figures are not presented in comparable form I am not at all sure of the accuracy of my inferences. In any case, there is so much in the way of historical development that is not covered that one cannot arrive at any relevant answer. It may be that the spread of commercial services in the United States was itself due to the failure of the voluntary services to supply enough blood, to give one simple hypothesis. The comparison might indeed indicate that the United States is a less altruistic society than the United Kingdom, but it would not show that commercial blood-giving was a cause rather than an effect.

In any case the empirical evidence can only be made meaningful with at least a minimum of theoretical analysis. *Why* should it be that the creation of a market for blood would decrease the altruism embodied in giving blood? I do not find any clear answer in Titmuss. He does make the following statement: "In not asking for or expecting any payment of money, these donors signify their belief in the willingness of other men to act altruistically in the future, and to combine together to make a gift freely available should they have a need for it. By expressing confidence in the behavior of future unknown strangers, they were thus denying the Hobbesian thesis that men are devoid of any distinctive moral sense" (p. 239). The statement does indeed imply that individuals will be willing to give without payment. But it does not explain why this willingness should be affected by the fact that other individuals receive money for these services, especially when the others include those whose need for financial reward is much greater. Evidently Titmuss must feel that attaching a price tag to this activity anywhere in the system depreciates its value as a symbolic expression of faith in others. But note that this is really an empirical question, not a matter of first principles. Do people in fact perceive the signals as Titmuss suggests? Would they, were the moral questions expounded with greater clarity?

II. GIVING AND EFFICIENCY

The aspect of Titmuss' work that will probably have the most striking effect both immediately and in the long run is his argument and evidence that a world of giving may actually increase efficiency in the operation of the economic system. This is on the face of it a dramatic challenge to the tenets of the mainstream of economic thought. Since the time of Adam Smith, economists have preached the virtues of the price system in enforcing efficiency and penalizing waste. To be sure, there has grown up a tradition, stemming from Alfred Marshall and developed by A. C. Pigou, Allyn Young, F. H. Knight, and more recent writers, which emphasizes that the price system does not always work satisfactorily. There are, in the language of welfare economics, "externalities," benefits and costs transmitted among individuals for which compensation in price terms is not and perhaps cannot be obtained. The problem of pollution has always been a standard example; the costs to others of the emission of noxious substances from smoke-stacks is not usually paid for. No self-enforcing price system would be feasible.

When we introduce externalities into the picture of resource allo-cation, we are really implying a very broad concept of efficiency. Effi-ciency is here measured with reference to a wide class of goods and evils, whether they are marketable or not. A system is inefficient if there is another way of allocating these goods, all the goods that we consider relevant, such that everybody is better off according to appro-priate criteria. These criteria might be clean air or the availability of blood when needed as well as automobiles or steak.

Titmuss presents a powerful indictment of the efficiency of blood-giving in the United States. The inefficiencies he finds are of three sorts: the imposition of unnecessary risks on recipients, the imposi-tion of unnecessary risks on certain classes of donors, and the preva-lence of waste and shortage in the distribution of blood.

With regard to the first, dramatic evidence has been advanced by Titmuss. The essential problem is that the use of infected blood in transfusions can lead to serum hepatitis in the recipient (as well as certain other diseases of much lower incidence). Not only Titmuss but a number of American investigators have shown that there is a remarkably high rate of post-transfusion serum hepatitis, an inci-dence which may reach 3 to 4 percent. Hepatitis is a serious illness and occasionally fatal. Out of those over age forty who receive trans-fusions, about one in one hundred and fifty die of it. Most striking of all, there seems to be very clear evidence that it is the commercial blood that is the primary source of hepatitis. Titmuss cites statistics showing that the risk of infection from blood given by prison and skid row populations is over ten times as great as from the population in general. One highly controlled study yielded very convincing evidence. The subjects underwent cardiac surgery, in which large amounts of blood were used, an average of eighteen to nineteen pints per person. Half the group was given blood from commercial sources, half from unpaid sources. The incidence of hepatitis in the first group was 53 percent, that in the second zero percent (the figure of 53 percent is not as far out of line with the 3 to 4 percent incidence as might be sup-posed; the eighteen or nineteen units of blood represent a corresponding number of individual opportunities to become infected, any one of which would suffice). On the other hand, the incidence of post-transfusion serum hepatitis in the United Kingdom is apparently less than 1 percent.

Further evidence comes from such comparisons as are possible with other countries. In West Germany, where evidently most of the blood is supplied commercially, post-transfusion hepatitis is estimated at 14 percent; in Japan, where virtually all the blood is commercial, the incidence is between 18 and 25 percent.[7]

The basic problem here is one that has many parallels. The commodity or service offered has uncertain characteristics. The buyer is not really in a position to know what it is that he is buying. In many circumstances buyers can protect themselves by testing the product in one way or another. If the product is one that is frequently used, then past experience can serve as a guide, particularly if the consequences of a defective performance are not especially severe. In other circumstances buyers are able to protect themselves by formal tests of not too great expense. This solution is unfortunately not available here. There is at the present time no test that can accurately detect whether a given blood donor is capable of transmitting hepatitis. The recently developed Au antigen test can detect only about 30 percent of potential infectors.

Now a situation in which the quality of a service is uncertain is not in itself an especially difficult situation to analyze. Every case of major surgery involves exactly the same considerations, the possibility of a large benefit weighed against some possibility of failure or even death. No doubt there are special considerations attached to high risk, but there is a further and very important distinction to be made in the case of blood donors. Usually the donor will know that he has had hepatitis, and therefore his truthfulness in recording his past history is of the utmost importance. At the same time, at least if the blood

7. According to such data as Titmuss could locate, commercial blood was very common in most countries and overwhelmingly so in the U.S.S.R., where about 50 percent of the blood is paid for at a very high rate. In Sweden, usually regarded as a society oriented toward collectivism, all of the blood is paid for. It is gathered by the state, not by commercial blood banks. The percentage of commercial blood in East Germany exceeds that in West Germany.

is to be collected in large quantities at relatively low cost, there is little or no opportunity to check the donor's word.

The situation is precisely the one alluded to earlier, that the virtue of truthfulness in fact contributes in a very significant way to the efficiency of the economic system. The supplying of truthful information is an example of an externality, if you like, but that classification does not really help us in deciding how truth is to be obtained. A voluntary donor system is from this point of view self-enforcing. Anyone whose motive for giving is to help others, but who suffers from hepatitis and is aware of the implications of this, will of course refrain from giving. On the other hand, a commercial blood donor, especially one driven by poverty, has every incentive to conceal the truth.

To repeat, the two key features of the situation are uncertainty about the quality of the service and a difference between the degrees of knowledge possessed by buyer and seller. The situation here is exacerbated by the severity of the risks involved. One can think of many parallels, and these have given rise to significant questions about the nature of responsibility in economic life. A good example is the question of automobile safety. The seller is supplying a complex machine. The details of both design and construction are inevitably better known to the seller than to the buyer. Further, if the risk of disastrous consequences is relatively low, no buyer can hope to acquire the relevant information from experience. In these circumstances it seems clear to me that the price system is no insurance of efficiency in all respects. The qualities of the product are simply not well defined from the buyer's point of view. Some alternative system of determining quality and providing assurance for buyers is needed. One such candidate is a sense of social responsibility on the part of the seller. This may indeed be easier to create in the case of the large organization than in that of the individual seller, for the obligation may then fall upon the individual members of that organization. In this context, ethical behavior can be regarded as a socially desirable institution which facilitates the achievement of economic efficiency in the broad sense.

I should add that, like many economists, I do not want to rely too heavily on substituting ethics for self-interest. I think it best on the whole that the requirement of ethical behavior be confined to those circumstances where the price system breaks down for the reasons suggested above. Wholesale usage of ethical standards is apt to have undesirable consequences. We do not wish to use up recklessly the scarce resources of altruistic motivation, and in any case ethically motivated behavior may even have a negative value to others if the agent acts without sufficient knowledge of the situation. In the case of medical practice and elsewhere, it might be plausibly argued that ethical codes serve as an instrument for increasing the economic advantage of one segment of the population at the expense of the rest.

It also appears that commercial blood-giving leads to unanticipated risks to the donors, though much less serious than those to the recipients. Commercial blood donors have some incentive to give blood more frequently than is desirable from the point of view of their health. This in and of itself is something of a gray area, because presumably the individual has some freedom of choice in such cases; but there is the possibility of a much more acute problem with respect to something like 20 percent of the blood collected. For many purposes, particularly the treatment of anemia, only the red blood cells are needed. There has been developed a new process called plasmapheresis. Here the red blood cells are separated from the plasma in which they float and the plasma is then reinjected into the body of the donor. Under these conditions donations can be, and are, made much more frequently. Several donations a week can be made, or so it is held. The collection of red blood cells for plasmapheresis is almost exclusively commercial, being carried out by or on behalf of the pharmaceutical companies. The fact that a very substantial income can be had through frequent donations means at least the potentiality of serious risk to the donors. There is, however, very little evidence of any damage actually having taken place.

A third apparent inefficiency in the United States system, according to Titmuss, is a very substantial amount of wastage of the blood collected; persistent shortages are also observed. Blood deteriorates after being drawn from a donor, and for most purposes it must be used within twenty-one days of collection. If the figures for collection and transfusion are compared, it appears that about 30 percent of the blood is wasted (the figures, as Titmuss notes, are far from adequate). Titmuss does not present any exactly comparable data for the United

Kingdom. If one compares the number of bottles "issued" with the number collected as given in one of his tables, there would seem to be about 10 percent wastage. However, there is a further possibility of wastage of bottles issued but not actually used in transfusions. The evidence for the existence of shortages is largely confined to several quotations from American authors (pp. 66-67). He notes that elective surgery is occasionally postponed because of the shortage of blood. It is asserted that no such shortages exist in the United Kingdom; a study by two economists that arrives at the opposite conclusion is abruptly dismissed by Titmuss as having been badly designed.[8] How supply and demand in the United Kingdom happened to balance so well over a period of twenty years in which the demand per capita has been rising steadily (due to new surgical techniques requiring much more blood) is left unexplained by Titmuss. Economists are accustomed to the idea of explaining the balance of supply and demand by the movement of prices. In the absence of prices something else must do the job. Perhaps there has been an expansion of the facilities for taking blood, but nothing in the book explains this remarkable parallel growth.

Although Titmuss links wastage of blood to the commercial system, he really gives no theoretical explanation of this link. I cannot conceive what it is. One would be much more tempted to explain a greater wastage of blood in the United States, if such exists, by the generally decentralized nature of the American blood collection system.[9] It should be noted that the voluntary system is quite chaotic as far as its organization is concerned. It is possible that, in the absence of a clear system of meeting shortages of a perishable commodity in one place with surpluses from another, such a system would perform much less efficiently than the British National Health Service. I find no clear evidence that commercialism per se is the key factor here.

In concluding this discussion of the relation between giving and efficiency, it strikes me that the essential point is the great importance of such a virtue as truthfulness in widely prevalent circumstances of

8. M. H. Cooper and A. J. Culyer, *The Price of Blood*, Hobart Paper No. 41, The Institute of Economic Affairs (London, 1968).

9. Just after these lines were written, President Nixon called for a study of the blood bank systems; the lack of coordination of the system was particularly noted (*New York Times*, 3 March 1972, p. 1).

economic life. I have remarked on the responsibility for truthfulness in economic life, but the issue goes even further. Virtually every commercial transaction has within itself an element of trust, certainly any transaction conducted over a period of time. It can be plausibly argued that much of the economic backwardness in the world can be explained by the lack of mutual confidence; see Banfield's remarkable study of a small community in southern Italy.[10]

I have considered the situation in which the quality of the commodity or service may be unknown to one side or the other in a transaction. It may also be that the price is unknown, that is, the price that could be commanded in some alternative market. Taking advantage of a situation where the other party in a transaction is ignorant of the potential price of a commodity or service might be regarded as a classic definition of "exploitation."

More basic yet, I will say, is the idea that the price system, in order to work at all, must involve the concept of property (even in the socialistic state there is public property). Property systems are in general not completely self-enforcing. They depend for their definition upon a constellation of legal procedures, both civil and criminal. The course of the law itself cannot be regarded as subject to the price system. The judges and the police may indeed be paid, but the system itself would disappear if on each occasion they were to sell their services and decisions. Thus the definition of property rights based on the price system depends precisely on the lack of universality of private property and of the price system. This ties in with the third hypothesis put forward in section I. The price system is not, and perhaps in some basic sense cannot be, universal. To the extent that it is incomplete, it must be supplemented by an implicit or explicit social contract. Thus one might loosely say that the categorical imperative and the price system are essential complements.

III. GIVING AND THE SOCIAL ORDER

Titmuss here and throughout his work is interested in still broader issues. For him the marketplace is basically subversive of the ideal social order. Some of his chapter titles are suggestive: "Blood and the

10. Edward C. Banfield, *The Moral Basis of a Backward Society* (New York, 1958).

Marketplace," "Economic Man: Social Man," and "Who is My
Stranger?" He appeals to Tönnies' familiar dichotomy between
Gemeinschaft and *Gesellschaft*. He greatly fears that "the myth of
maximizing economic growth can supplant the growth of economic
social relation" (p. 199).[11]

It is worthwhile to summarize a genuinely horrifying case which
serves Titmuss as an empirical springboard for his general attack on
the commercialization of society. In the mid-1950's the blood supply
in Kansas City was essentially completely in the hands of commercial
blood banks, whose quality is described as very unsatisfactory. As a
result a community blood bank was organized on a volunteer basis,
and the hospitals insisted on drawing their blood only from this
source. The commercial blood banks attacked the hospitals for violation of the antitrust laws, and after long and expensive testimony
before the Federal Trade Commission the hospitals were forbidden to
discriminate against commercial blood. It should, however, be added
that this decision was subsequently overturned by the courts.

The key issue here as Titmuss sees it is the fact that this case was
regarded as subject to the antitrust laws because blood was treated
as a commodity. It is the latter point that disturbs Titmuss and
arouses his ire. He generalizes from this to the whole treatment of
medical care as a commodity. He notes, with appropriate statistics,
that malpractice suits have become increasingly prevalent in the
United States. The cost of malpractice insurance is rising, the settle-
ments are growing in size as well as in number. All this is contrasted
with the British situation, in which malpractice suits are apparently
quite negligible in number and seriousness. What do these observa-
tions in fact tell us? Titmuss, without giving a detailed theoretical
explanation, suggests in a general sort of way that the commercializa-

11. His antagonism to at least some economists is stated strongly a few lines
below this quotation. "In saying this we recall that Keynes once expressed the
hope that one day economists 'could manage to get themselves thought of as
competent people on a level with dentists.' This day has not yet dawned for some
of the order who, after taking strong oaths of ethical neutrality, perform as mis-
sionaries in the social welfare field and often give the impression of possessively
owning a hot line to God." The reference is clearly to those laissez faire economists, of whom there is an organized group in the United Kingdom, who have
favored placing the blood supply and indeed the whole medical system in private
hands.

tion of medical practice is accompanied by a legitimization of doctor-patient hostility.

One can, it seems to me, look at this matter somewhat differently. The ideal of Titmuss could be interpreted as that of a world where doctors and hospitals are protected from the consequences of their errors, at least as far as legal proceedings are concerned. After all, there is one very important relevant question: Are the malpractice suits justified? I have no reason to believe that the courts have any biases against physicians. If anything, one would suppose the opposite. There may conceivably be biases in the procedure as such, but these have not been demonstrated, and in the absence of evidence to the contrary I think we can trust the courts to have made a much more detailed inquiry in each case than the social scientist can do. If this is so, then we have to reckon with the idea that there is a lot of malpractice in the United States. To discourage suits, then, would simply be a way of denying compensation to legitimate victims for the costs imposed upon them, and of minimizing a method of exerting pressure on doctors who perform badly. Titmuss views the latter contingency positively. He refers to the increased costs due to what is frequently termed defensive practice, the excess of precautions necessary to prevent future claims of malpractice; but after all, it may well be true that a little more care might be good rather than bad. In any case, the assertion that malpractice suits induce excessive care rather than better care should not be presumed sound without further evidence.

Titmuss quite candidly agrees that there may well be trouble with patients' claims in the United Kingdom: "All in all, the scales are weighted in favor of the doctor" (p. 170). He urges that there are remedies other than litigation but does not specify them. What is disturbing, in this case as in many others, is that an appeal against the marketplace and its coldness has a way of slipping into a defense of privilege. The *Gemeinschaft-Gesellschaft* dichotomy can be couched in different language; Maine spoke of the difference between status and contract.[12] It is very easy indeed for "community" to slip over into "status."

12. Henry Maine, *Ancient Law* (London, 1861).

Indeed, there is something of a paradox in Titmuss' philosophy. He is especially interested in the expression of impersonal altruism. It is not the richness of family relationships or the close ties of a small community that he wishes to promote. It is rather a diffuse expression of confidence by individuals in the workings of a society as a whole. But such an expression of impersonal altruism is as far removed from the feelings of personal interaction as any marketplace. Indeed, the small number of blood donors in the United Kingdom suggests, if I were to generalize as freely as Titmuss does, the idea of an aristocracy of saints. I suppose this idea is indeed in the Fabian tradition; at any rate, it is certainly expressed with great clarity by Shaw in *Man and Superman*. This is a way of social life that seems to have worked remarkably well in the British context, while proving capable of catastrophic consequences in the Soviet Union.

The pervasive fear in Titmuss' thinking that commercialism may increasingly damage the entire social system is in many curious ways a mirror image of Hayek's.[13] Hayek and Titmuss seem to agree that a mixed economy is necessarily unstable. But whereas Hayek believes that a little bit of collectivism is likely to lead to a total dictatorship, Titmuss is concerned rather with the insidious nature of a price system. Both arguments have a resemblance to some of those connected with abortion. If you allow abortion, how can you argue against homicide?

The first thing about the argument of instability is that it is, after all, strictly an empirical one. It simply may not be true. It is very hard to believe that the use of commercial blood in the United States has any important effect on the general doctor-patient relationship. That relation is governed essentially by the same principles as always; if anything, the spread of medical insurance has weakened rather than strengthened the commercial link between doctor and patient. In the United Kingdom, of course, the relation is different, but I wonder if malpractice suits were any more common in the period before the National Health Service was instituted.

The second difficulty with this argument is that it has a rather elitist flavor. Presumably, the high value of altruism or whatever other virtue is threatened by the growth of commercialization will still hold

13. Friedrich A. Hayek, *The Road to Serfdom* (Chicago and London, 1944).

even after the price system has spread somewhat. What Titmuss would be afraid of, I take it, is that other, weaker souls would somehow succumb. In the present context, perhaps individuals will cease to give blood when they see that other people are being paid for it. Now, the argument that we should therefore not permit a commercial system amounts to saying both that I am more foresighted than my contemporaries and that my virtue is less assailable. Perhaps these propositions are really true, but I find them at any rate uncomfortable.

IV. REMARKS ON EMPIRICAL VALIDITY

At the beginning of this discussion I quoted Titmuss' final paragraphs, a statement which embodies a remarkably large number of empirical conclusions. It cannot really be maintained that most of them have been established. The most dramatic and best sustained is unquestionably the relation between the commercial blood supply and post-transfusion hepatitis. This indictment alone is fully worth the entire investigation. The evidences of inefficiency in the United States are also clear, though I find their causes less well established.

Indeed, with respect to empirical methodology there is much to be desired. Titmuss gives no consideration to the role of theory in empirical research. He seems to regard the argument *post hoc, ergo propter hoc* as infallible. At any rate, in most instances the comparisons used involve two cases between which there are many differences. The commercialization of the blood supply can certainly not have all the consequences that he apparently ascribes to it.

Even by the least stringent rules for evaluating empirical evidence, many of Titmuss' points are not in any way established. I see, for example, no real evidence that the presence of a commercial blood supply decreases the amount of altruism. This is not to say that it may not do so; but the data for the two countries is not presented in forms sufficiently comparable to allow any statement whatever. Compensating factors are never considered; thus the point Titmuss makes about the redistribution of blood from the poor to the rich is not in any way offset by the fact of a corresponding flow of money from the rich to the poor, a point which should at least be taken into consideration.

Despite Titmuss' careful use of data in some places, he is very loose in others. On several less important points he makes statements about the United States without even bothering to compare the situation with that in the United Kingdom, although without such comparison there is no evidence of any kind. For example, as an evidence of the shortage of blood in the United States he observes that if hemophiliacs were given blood without restraint they would consume an amount equal to one-eighth of the blood used in the United States. Presumably the incidence of hemophilia is the same in the United Kingdom as in the United States, yet Titmuss does not bother to tell us whether hemophiliacs are in fact treated as fully there as he would have them treated here.

Again, as evidence of the corruption introduced into the United States medical system by commercialization he includes several damaging anecdotes about unethical medical experiments. No statement whatever is made about the ethics of experimentation in the United Kingdom. In fact, the United States today probably has the most stringent rules regarding such practices of any country in the world, requiring informed consent of the subject. Finally, for all Titmuss' strictures on the dangers involved in plasmapheresis, he does not have anything to say about this practice in the United Kingdom. Possibly it is unknown there, but the book is not clear on this point.

Despite—and in part because of—its flaws, Titmuss' book is a resonant evocation of central problems of social value. His blithe disregard of the usual epistemological strictures against confusion of act and value permits him to raise the largest descriptive and normative questions about the social order in a highly specific and richly factual context. This is not a systematic, abstract work on the foundations of ethics. It is not a meticulous descriptive and causal analysis of the functioning of social systems. But by suggestively combining a passionately informed commitment to an ideal social order and an illustration of problems within the context of a concrete situation, it has greatly enriched the quality of social-philosophical debate.

PETER SINGER

Altruism and Commerce:
A Defense of
Titmuss against Arrow

Kenneth Arrow's discussion[1] of *The Gift Relationship* by Richard Titmuss[2] is to be welcomed because it draws attention to this remarkable book. Ostensibly, the book is a comparison of voluntary and commercial means of obtaining blood for medical purposes, but by means of this comparison Titmuss succeeds, as Arrow says, in raising "the largest descriptive and normative questions about the social order in a highly specific and richly factual context" (p. 158). Although Arrow praises the endeavor, he is not very keen on what Titmuss actually says about these issues. I wish to defend Titmuss against some of Arrow's criticisms.

First, there are some minor points on which Arrow does not appear to have read Titmuss with sufficient care. Twice Arrow claims that Titmuss, though critical of particular aspects of the United States blood supply system, fails to indicate whether the situation is different under the fully voluntary British system (pp. 157-158). In fact, Titmuss does make the comparison both times, once quite explicitly, and once implicitly.[3] Then, after noting the evidence Titmuss gives that there is far greater wastage of blood (a perishable commodity) in the American system, Arrow states that no theoretical explanation of the link between wastage and a commercial system of obtaining blood is given, and that he, Arrow, cannot conceive what the link

1. "Gifts and Exchanges," *Philosophy & Public Affairs* I, no. 4 (Summer 1972): 343-362, and above, pp. 139-158. All otherwise unidentified page references are to this article.
2. (London and New York, 1971.)
3. *The Gift Relationship*, pp. 206-207 and 23.

could be (p. 152). Titmuss does offer an explanation: because blood is perishable, efficiency depends on a regular and predictable source of supply, and commercial systems tend to pick up a much higher percentage of irregular "Skid Row" types than do voluntary systems.[4] This explanation may not be accepted, but it should at least be recognized that one has been offered.

The first major criticism Arrow makes concerns the view, advanced by Titmuss, that the introduction of "the laws of the marketplace" into an area like the supply of blood means that men are no longer able to give their blood freely and altruistically. Instead, Titmuss says, they are "coerced and constrained by the market." By contrast, in a voluntary system donors "signify their belief in the willingness of other men to act altruistically in the future and to combine together to make a gift freely available should they have a need for it."[5]

Arrow, on the other hand, defends the economists' assumption that "since the creation of a market increases the individual's area of choice it therefore leads to higher benefits." The existence of a commercial system in addition to a voluntary one, according to orthodox economic ideas, gives everyone the freedom to choose whether to sell their blood or donate it freely. It does not impair anyone's right to give; it merely provides an alternative if it should be wanted. Against Titmuss's claim that we must choose between the freedom of the marketplace and the freedom to give altruistically, Arrow says: "I can find no support in the evidence for the existence of such a dilemma. Indeed, it is not easy to see what kind of evidence would be relevant" (p. 146).

Perhaps the way in which Titmuss puts the dilemma is misleading. To talk as if the choice is between incompatible *freedoms*, or between a "right to give" and a "right to sell," seems a distortion of the language of freedom and rights. If Arrow had limited himself to pointing out that we are still *free* to give even when others are selling blood, that we can still exercise the right to give *if* we choose to do so, one could agree with him. Even if the issue is not one of choosing between incompatible freedoms, however, there remains a real dilemma; for what Titmuss is really asserting is that a voluntary system fosters attitudes of altruism and a desire to relate to, and help,

4. *Ibid.*, p. 22.   5. *Ibid.*, p. 239.

strangers in one's community. While a voluntary system, Titmuss alleges, fosters these attitudes and creates opportunities for their expression, a commercial system would have the opposite effect. The laws of the marketplace discourage altruism and fellow-feeling. Even if the opportunity to give still existed, the attitude toward giving would no longer be the same.[6]

It is with regard to this latter claim, as well as the formulation of the dilemma in terms of a choice between freedoms, that Arrow finds "no support in the evidence."

The extent to which it is reasonable to demand conclusive or very strong evidence before a proposition is taken seriously must vary with the nature of the proposition that is being considered. In a case like the comparison of blood supply systems in different countries, where controlled experiments are impossible and the factor under examination can never be isolated from other differences between the systems, it is unreasonable to demand conclusive proof or anything near it. *Some* genuine evidence there must of course be, before we accept, even tentatively, the view that a commercial system discourages altruism; but once there is some evidence, the onus is on whoever denies this to produce counterevidence.

Evidence of this sort, inconclusive but still significant, is to be found in *The Gift Relationship*. It consists, first, in the contrasting trends to be found in the statistics on voluntary donors in England and Wales, on the one hand, and in the United States and Japan on the other; and second, in the statements of the British voluntary donors themselves. A brief account of this evidence follows.

The demand for blood has risen sharply in recent years, partly as a result of new surgery techniques, partly for social and economic reasons. In England and Wales, where all donors are unpaid, the number of donations has increased sufficiently to cover this increased demand. Since 1948, when the National Health Service was introduced, and 1968, the number of donations has increased by 277 percent; and between 1961 and 1967 (a period chosen for comparative purposes) the increase was 31 percent.[7] Thanks to the increase in volunteers, Titmuss tells us, the National Blood Transfusion Board

6. Titmuss has confirmed this interpretation in a private communication.
7. *The Gift Relationship*, pp. 42-43.

"has never consciously been aware of a shortage, or an impending shortage of potential donors."[8] Over the same period from 1961 to 1967 in the United States, on the other hand, while commercial banks and community banks with over 50 percent paid donors collected increased supplies, the number of units of blood collected from other banks, relying mainly on unpaid donors, actually fell.[9] (By 1967, only 9 percent of United States donors were truly voluntary.) In New York, the only city to have published sufficient figures to indicate a trend, voluntary community donations fell from 20 percent of total supplies in 1956 to 1 percent in 1966.[10] The rise in commercial supplies has not been sufficient to compensate for the fall in unpaid donations and to cope as well with the increased demand; the consequence has been serious shortages.[11]

In Japan, the decline in unpaid donors has been even more acute. Prior to 1951, apparently, donors were not paid, but at that time the need to supply blood to American forces in Korea led to the introduction of payment. Now 98 percent of all blood is paid for, and the shortage of blood is said to be still more critical than in the United States.[12]

The overall picture, then, is that where payment for blood is unknown, the number of voluntary donors has risen and kept pace with the increased demand; whereas when the opportunity to give freely exists alongside the buying and selling of blood, the number of volunteers falls sharply and can only with difficulty, if at all, be made good by increases in the amount of blood bought. This suggests that to pay some people for their blood does discourage others from giving it altruistically; or alternatively, that a purely voluntary system encourages altruism in a way that a mixed commercial-voluntary system does not.

Arrow demands not merely evidence, but (p. 147) "at least a minimum of theoretical analysis. *Why* should it be that the creation of a market for blood would decrease the altruism embodied in giving blood?" The second kind of evidence to be found in *The Gift Relationship* is concerned with the motivation of voluntary donors in Britain. As such, it may help us to understand the connection between

8. *Ibid.*, p. 120.   9. *Ibid.*, p. 59.   10. *Ibid.*, p. 96.
11. *Ibid.*, pp. 39-40.   12. *Ibid.*, p. 156.

altruism and the voluntary system while at the same time supporting
the claim that there is such a connection.

This evidence comes from a questionnaire survey of blood donors
in England taken by Titmuss and his associates.[13] One question asked
was: "Could you say why you *first* decided to become a blood donor?"
Statistically, all that can be said is that nearly 80 percent of the 3,800
answers Titmuss collected indicate that the respondent was motivated
by a high sense of social responsibility toward the needs of others. It
is true that these people might have continued to give blood unpaid,
and for the same reasons, even if a commercial system existed along
with the voluntary one; but it is worth noting (although no statistical
significance is being claimed here) that at least some of the answers
do suggest a connection between the special status of blood under
the voluntary system, and the motivation of the donors. For instance,
a young married woman, a machine operator earning £15 to £20 per
week, replied:

> You cant get blood from supermarkets and chaine stores. People
> them selves must come forword, sick people cant get out of bed to
> ask you for a pint to save thier life so I came forword in hope to
> help somebody who needs blood.

Despite her obvious lack of education, this woman expressed the
essential point Titmuss is making: in Britain the supply of blood is
outside the otherwise pervasive supermarket society. No matter how
much money you have, you can't buy yourself a pint of blood. You
must rely on the altruism and good will of others to provide it for you.
Once commercial blood supplies are introduced, even though the voluntary system may continue to operate as well, this situation has been
altered. Provided you have money, you do not then need the altruism
of your fellow men and women, since you can buy the blood you need.
So commerce replaces fellow-feeling. Marx was well aware of this
effect of commerce, and described it vividly:

> The extent of the power of money is the extent of my power.
> Money's properties are my properties and essential powers—the
> properties and powers of its possessor. Thus what I am and am

13. *Ibid.*, pp. 226-235, 276-320.

capable of is by no means determined by my individuality. I am ugly, but I can buy for myself the most beautiful of women. Therefore I am not ugly for the effect of ugliness—its deterrent power—is nullified by money. . . . That which I am unable to do as a *man* . . . I am able to do by means of *money*. . . . Money, then, appears as this overturning power both against the individual and against the bonds of society. . . . Assume *man* to be *man* and his relationship to the world to be a human one: then you can exchange love only for love, trust for trust, etc.[14]

We do not, however, need to go into the Marxist theory of money as an alienating force in order to understand how a voluntary blood supply system—or more generally, a system of free medicine like the British National Health Service—may strengthen feelings of community and mutual interdependence. I think it is clear that the woman whose reply has been quoted would have been less likely to give her blood if blood were a marketable commodity. Some of the other responses to Titmuss's questionnaire indicate this in different, though equally direct, ways:

I get my surgical shoes thro' the N.H.S. This is some slight return and I want to help people (an insurance agent).

To try and repay in some small way some unknown person whose blood helped me recover from two operations and enable me to be with my family, thats why I bring them along also as they become old enough (a farmer's wife).

No man is an island (a maintenance fitter).[15]

14. Karl Marx, *The Economic and Philosophic Manuscripts of 1844*, trans. M. Milligan, ed. D. J. Struik (New York, 1967), pp. 167-169. (For more on the same theme, see also the section entitled "The Power of Money in Bourgeois Society.") I think this quotation shows that Titmuss himself is unfair to Marx when he relates the commercially minded attitude to blood supplies in the Soviet Union to Marx's theory of the commodity (*The Gift Relationship*, p. 195).

15. *The Gift Relationship*, pp. 227-228. In discussing the percentage of British donors who are fully voluntary, Arrow notes that in the case of 28 percent of British donors either they or their family have received blood transfusions (p. 347). Since this remark follows immediately on the comment that Titmuss has not classified British donors in a manner comparable to his classification of United States donors, it implies that Arrow would put these British donors into

The nature of these replies—not the mere fact that the donors were altruistically motivated, but their attitudes toward the National Health Service in general and the Blood Transfusion Service in particular—is evidence that at least for some people the possibility of others buying and selling blood would destroy the inspiring force behind their own donations. At the same time, these replies enable us to understand *why* the existence of a commercial system could be expected to make a difference. The idea that others are depending on one's generosity and concern, that one may oneself, in an emergency, need the assistance of a stranger, the feeling that there is still at least this vital area in which we must rely on the good will of others rather than the profit motive—all these vague ideas and feelings are incompatible with the existence of a market in blood. Do we really need any further "theoretical analysis"?

Arrow is critical of Titmuss for favoring the voluntary system on broad grounds of principle, unsupported by adequate statistical evidence. Yet Arrow has his own opposite preferences, at least equally unsupported. Arrow frankly admits that:

> . . . like many economists, I do not want to rely too heavily on substituting ethics for self-interest. I think it best on the whole that the requirement of ethical behavior be confined to those circumstances where the price system breaks down. . . . Wholesale usage of ethical standards is apt to have undesirable consequences. We do not wish to use up recklessly the scarce resources of altruistic motivation . . . (pp. 150-151).

---

the same category as those in the United States who are replacing blood received by themselves or their relatives, and whom Titmuss does not count as fully voluntary. This seems to be another oversight on Arrow's part. Titmuss does classify British donors in exactly the same terms as United States donors, and concludes that 99 percent—all but the donations of prisoners, who may be under some external pressure—are fully voluntary (*The Gift Relationship*, p. 130). The point is that in Britain people who need blood get it irrespective of whether they have given blood, or undertake to give it in the future; in the United States various schemes exist under which unpaid donations either replace blood received that would otherwise have to be paid for, or are a form of credit in case one needs blood in the future. This is why "reciprocal" donations in the United States could have a purely self-interested motivation, whereas in Britain they are a sign of community feeling.

Arrow offers no evidence or theory for the view that altruism resembles, say, oil in being a scarce resource, the more of which we use the less we have. Why should we not assume that altruism is more like sexual potency—much used, it constantly renews itself, but if rarely called upon, it will be begin to atrophy and will not be available when needed? It is this latter simile which consideration of my own feelings leads me to favor. I find it hardest to act with consideration for others when the norm in the circle of people I move in is to act egoistically. When altruism is expected of me, however, I find it much easier to be genuinely altruistic.

Indeed, there is experimental evidence for the view that altruism fosters increased altruism. Psychologists have found that if they set up situations calling for an altruistic response—for example, a woman looking helpless beside a broken-down car—more people will respond with offers of help if they have recently witnessed someone else behaving altruistically in a similar situation (i.e., because the experimenters put a man helping a woman to change a tire back down the road) than if they had not witnessed an altruistic act.[16] These results, hardly surprising results really, give some support to Titmuss's view that the opportunity for altruism promotes further altruism, and count against the idea that altruism is a finite resource.

Finally, I would like to touch upon an important theoretical issue raised by *The Gift Relationship* which Arrow did not really discuss. Can economic analysis be value free? The whole approach Titmuss takes to the particular subject of blood supply systems is based on the conviction that it cannot be. Titmuss disputes the claims of "value-free" economics because he is concerned to defend Britain's voluntary system against criticisms by right-wing economists who purport to show the superiority of the commercial system on purely economic grounds. In a study called *The Price of Blood* commissioned by the Institute of Economic Affairs,[17] the authors maintain that "the simplest tools of economic analysis" support the view that human blood

16. A summary of this and other experiments along similar lines may be found in D. Wright, *The Psychology of Moral Behavior* (London and Baltimore, 1971), pp. 133-139.

17. M. H. Cooper and A. J. Culyer, *The Price of Blood* (London, 1968); cited by Titmuss in *The Gift Relationship*, p. 195.

is an economic good and that a commercial system is superior on purely economic grounds.

Titmuss refutes this view on its own terms before challenging the whole approach to the topic. He is able to show that the cost per unit of blood is between five and fifteen times higher in the United States than in Britain; moreover this blood is much more likely to be contaminated and infect the recipient with hepatitis. All this can be demonstrated without raising questions of values. What cannot be demonstrated in this way, and what therefore put limits to the scope of value-free economics, are the social utilities involved in the possibilities for altruistic behavior which are lost when economic relations are substituted for voluntary donations. Here we must ask ourselves not "How can we obtain the most blood at the least cost?" but "What sort of society do we want?" No value-free science can answer this question; at the same time, no investigation into the economics of methods of obtaining blood which, by ignoring the larger issue, gives the impression that these social utilities don't matter or are not relevant, can claim to be value free. Even if it is true that we do not have sufficient evidence to allow us to regard the connection between methods of obtaining blood and social attitudes of altruism as definitely established, this does not allow us legitimately to disregard any such connection for the purpose of recommending, say, the creation of a commercial system alongside a voluntary one. For to disregard such a connection would be to assume that none exists; and at the very least, the evidence Titmuss has produced gives rise to a presumption that there is some connection. Unless this presumption is rebutted, the nature of a community's blood supply cannot be considered a purely economic issue.

STEPHEN P. STICH   The Recombinant
                          DNA Debate

The debate over recombinant DNA research is a unique event, perhaps
a turning point, in the history of science. For the first time in modern
history there has been widespread public discussion about whether
and how a promising though potentially dangerous line of research
shall be pursued. At root the debate is a moral debate and, like most
such debates, requires proper assessment of the facts at crucial stages
in the argument. A good deal of the controversy over recombinant
DNA research arises because some of the facts simply are not yet
known. There are many empirical questions we would like to have
answered before coming to a decision—questions about the reliability
of proposed containment facilities, about the viability of enfeebled
strains of E. coli, about the ways in which pathogenic organisms do
their unwelcome work, and much more. But all decisions cannot wait
until the facts are available; some must be made now. It is to be expected that people with different hunches about what the facts will
turn out to be will urge different decisions on how recombinant DNA
research should be regulated. However, differing expectations about
the facts have not been the only fuel for controversy. A significant part
of the current debate can be traced to differences over moral principles. Also, unfortunately, there has been much unnecessary debate
generated by careless moral reasoning and a failure to attend to the
logical structure of some of the moral arguments that have been
advanced.

In order to help sharpen our perception of the moral issues underlying the controversy over recombinant DNA research, I shall start by clearing away some frivolous arguments that have deflected attention from more serious issues. We may then examine the problems involved in deciding whether the potential benefits of recombinant DNA research justify pursuing it despite the risks that it poses.

I. THREE BAD ARGUMENTS

My focus in this section will be on three untenable arguments, each of which has surfaced with considerable frequency in the public debate over recombinant DNA research.

The first argument on my list concludes that recombinant DNA research should not be controlled or restricted. The central premise of the argument is that scientists should have full and unqualified freedom to pursue whatever inquiries they may choose to pursue. This claim was stated repeatedly in petitions and letters to the editor during the height of the public debate over recombinant DNA research in the University of Michigan community.[1] The general moral principle which is the central premise of the argument plainly does entail that investigators using recombinant DNA technology should be allowed to pursue their research as they see fit. However, we need only consider a few examples to see that the principle invoked in this "freedom of inquiry" argument is utterly indefensible. No matter how sincere a researcher's interest may be in investigating the conjugal

1. For example, from a widely circulated petition signed by both faculty and community people: "The most important challenge may be a confrontation with one of our ancient assumptions—that there must be an absolute and unqualified freedom to pursue scientific inquiries. We will soon begin to wonder what meaning this freedom has if it leads to the destruction or demoralization of human beings, the only life forms able to exercise it." And from a letter to the editor written by a Professor of Engineering Humanities: "Is science beyond social and human controls, so that freedom of inquiry implies the absence of usual social restrictions which we all, as citizens, obey, respecting the social contract?"

It is interesting to note that the "freedom of inquiry" argument is rarely proposed by defenders of recombinant DNA research. Rather, it is proposed, then attacked, by those who are opposed to research involving recombinant molecules. Their motivation, it would seem, is to discredit the proponents of recombinant DNA research by attributing a foolish argument to them, then demonstrating that it is indeed a foolish argument.

behavior of American university professors, few would be willing to grant him the right to pursue his research in my bedroom without my consent. No matter how interested a researcher may be in investigating the effects of massive doses of bomb-grade plutonium on preschool children, it is hard to imagine that anyone thinks he should be allowed to do so. Yet the "free inquiry" principle, if accepted, would allow both of these projects and countless other Dr. Strangelove projects as well. So plainly the simplistic "free inquiry" principle is indefensible. It would, however, be a mistake to conclude that freedom of inquiry ought not to be protected. A better conclusion is that the right of free inquiry is a qualified right and must sometimes yield to conflicting rights and to the demands of conflicting moral principles. Articulating an explicit and properly qualified principle of free inquiry is a task of no small difficulty. We will touch on this topic again toward the end of Section II.

The second argument I want to examine aims at establishing just the opposite conclusion from the first. The particular moral judgment being defended is that there should be a total ban on recombinant DNA research. The argument begins with the observation that even in so-called low-risk recombinant DNA experiments there is at least a possibility of catastrophic consequences. We are, after all, dealing with a relatively new and unexplored technology. Thus it is at least possible that a bacterial culture whose genetic makeup has been altered in the course of a recombinant DNA experiment may exhibit completely unexpected pathogenic characteristics. Indeed, it is not impossible that we could find ourselves confronted with a killer strain of, say, *E. coli* and, worse, a strain against which humans can marshal no natural defense. Now if this is possible—if we cannot say with assurance that the probability of it happening is zero—then, the argument continues, all recombinant DNA research should be halted. For the negative utility of the imagined catastrophe is so enormous, resulting as it would in the destruction of our society and perhaps even of our species, that no work which could possibly lead to this result would be worth the risk.

The argument just sketched, which might be called the "doomsday scenario" argument, begins with a premise which no informed person would be inclined to deny. It is indeed *possible* that even a low-risk recombinant DNA experiment might lead to totally catastrophic results. No ironclad guarantee can be offered that this will not happen. And while the probability of such an unanticipated catastrophe is surely not large, there is no serious argument that the probability is zero. Still, I think the argument is a sophistry. To go from the undeniable premise that recombinant DNA research might possibly result in unthinkable catastrophe to the conclusion that such research should be banned requires a moral principle stating that *all* endeavors that might possibly result in such a catastrophe should be prohibited. Once the principle has been stated, it is hard to believe that anyone would take it at all seriously. For the principle entails that, along with recombinant DNA research, almost all scientific research and many other commonplace activities having little to do with science should be prohibited. It is, after all, at least logically possible that the next new compound synthesized in an ongoing chemical research program will turn out to be an uncontainable carcinogen many orders of magnitude more dangerous than aerosol plutonium. And, to vary the example, there is a non-zero probability that experiments in artificial pollination will produce a weed that will, a decade from now, ruin the world's food grain harvest.[2]

I cannot resist noting that the principle invoked in the doomsday scenario argument is not new. Pascal used an entirely parallel argument to show that it is in our own best interests to believe in God. For though the probability of God's existence may be very low, if He nonetheless should happen to exist, the disutility that would accrue to the disbeliever would be catastrophic—an eternity in hell. But, as introductory philosophy students should all know, Pascal's argument only looks persuasive if we take our options to be just two: Christianity

---

2. Unfortunately, the doomsday scenario argument is *not* a straw man conjured only by those who would refute it. Consider, for example, the remarks of Anthony Mazzocchi, spokesman for the Oil, Chemical and Atomic Workers International Union, reported in *Science News*, 19 March 1977, p. 181: "When scientists argue over safe or unsafe, we ought to be very prudent. . . . If critics are correct and the Andromeda scenario has *even the smallest possibility* of occurring, we must assume it will occur on the basis of our experience" (emphasis added).

or atheism. A third possibility is belief in a jealous non-Christian God who will see to our damnation if and only if we *are* Christians. The probability of such a deity existing is again very small, but non-zero. So Pascal's argument is of no help in deciding whether or not to accept Christianity. For we may be damned if we do and damned if we don't.

I mention Pascal's difficulty because there is a direct parallel in the doomsday scenario argument against recombinant DNA research. Just as there is a non-zero probability that unforeseen consequences of recombinant DNA research will lead to disaster, so there is a non-zero probability that unforeseen consequences of *failing* to pursue the research will lead to disaster. There may, for example, come a time when, because of natural or man-induced climatic change, the capacity to alter quickly the genetic constitution of agricultural plants will be necessary to forestall catastrophic famine. And if we fail to pursue recombinant DNA research now, our lack of knowledge in the future may have consequences as dire as any foreseen in the doomsday scenario argument.

The third argument I want to consider provides a striking illustration of how important it is, in normative thinking, to make clear the moral *principles* being invoked. The argument I have in mind begins with a factual claim about recombinant DNA research and concludes that stringent restrictions, perhaps even a moratorium, should be imposed. However, advocates of the argument are generally silent on the normative principle(s) linking premise and conclusion. The gap thus created can be filled in a variety of ways, resulting in very different arguments. The empirical observation that begins the argument is that recombinant DNA methods enable scientists to move genes back and forth across natural barriers, "particularly the most fundamental such barrier, that which divides prokaryotes from eukaryotes. The results will be essentially new organisms, self-perpetuating and hence permanent."[3] Because of this, it is concluded that severe restrictions are

3. The quotation is from George Wald, "The Case Against Genetic Engineering," *The Sciences*, September/October 1976; reprinted in David A. Jackson and Stephen P. Stich, eds., *The Recombinant DNA Debate* (Englewood Cliffs, N.J.: Prentice-Hall, 1979).

in order. Plainly this argument is an enthymeme; a central premise has been left unstated. What sort of moral principle is being tacitly assumed?

The principle that comes first to mind is simply that natural barriers should not be breached, or perhaps that "essentially new organisms" should not be created. The principle has an almost theological ring to it, and perhaps there are some people who would be prepared to defend it on theological grounds. But short of a theological argument, it is hard to see why anyone would hold the view that breaching natural barriers or creating new organisms is *intrinsically* wrong. For if a person were to advocate such a principle, he would have to condemn the creation of new bacterial strains capable of, say, synthesizing human clotting factor or insulin, *even if* creating the new organism generated *no unwelcome side effects.*

There is quite a different way of unraveling the "natural barriers" argument which avoids appeal to the dubious principles just discussed. As an alternative, this second reading of the argument ties premise to conclusion with a second factual claim and a quite different normative premise. The added factual claim is that at present our knowledge of the consequences of creating new forms of life is severely limited; thus we cannot know with any assurance that the probability of disastrous consequences is very low. The moral principle needed to mesh with the two factual premises would be something such as the following:

> If we do not know with considerable assurance that the probability of an activity leading to disastrous consequences is very low, then we should not allow the activity to continue.

Now this principle, unlike those marshaled in the first interpretation of the natural barriers argument, is not lightly dismissed. It is, to be sure, a conservative principle, and it has the odd feature of focusing entirely on the dangers an activity poses while ignoring its potential benefits.[4] Still, the principle may have a certain attraction in light of

4. It is important to note, however, that the principle is considerably less conservative, and correspondingly more plausible, than the principle invoked in the doomsday scenario argument. That latter principle would have us enjoin an activity if the probability of the activity leading to catastrophe is anything other than zero.

recent history, which has increasingly been marked by catastrophes attributable to technology's unanticipated side effects. I will not attempt a full scale evaluation of this principle just now. For the principle raises, albeit in a rather extreme way, the question of how risks and benefits are to be weighed against each other. In my opinion, that is the really crucial moral question raised by recombinant DNA research. It is a question which bristles with problems. In Section II I shall take a look at some of these problems and make a few tentative steps toward some solutions. While picking our way through the problems we will have another opportunity to examine the principle just cited.

II. RISKS AND BENEFITS

At first glance it might be thought that the issue of risks and benefits is quite straightforward, at least in principle. What we want to know is whether the potential benefits of recombinant DNA research justify the risks involved. To find out we need only determine the probabilities of the various dangers and benefits. And while some of the empirical facts—the probabilities—may require considerable ingenuity and effort to uncover, the assessment poses no particularly difficult normative or conceptual problems. Unfortunately, this sanguine view does not survive much more than a first glance. A closer look at the task of balancing the risks and benefits of recombinant DNA research reveals a quagmire of sticky conceptual problems and simmering moral disputes. In the next few pages I will try to catalogue and comment on some of these moral disputes. I wish I could also promise solutions to all of them, but to do so would be false advertising.

Problems about Probabilities

In trying to assess costs and benefits, a familiar first step is to set down a list of possible actions and possible outcomes. Next, we assign some measure of desirability to each possible outcome, and for each action we estimate the conditional probability of each outcome given that the action is performed. In attempting to apply this decision-making strategy to the case of recombinant DNA research, the assignment of probabilities poses some perplexing problems. Some of the outcomes whose probabilities we want to know can be approached using standard empirical techniques. Thus, for example, we may want to know what the probability is of a specific enfeebled host *E. coli* strain surviving passage through the human intestinal system, should it be accidentally ingested. Or we may want to know what the probability is that a host organism will escape from a P-4 laboratory. In such cases, while there may be technical difficulties to be overcome, we have a reasonably clear idea of the sort of data needed to estimate the required probabilities. But there are other possible outcomes whose probabilities cannot be determined by experiment. It is important, for example, to know what the probability is of recombinant DNA research leading to a method for developing nitrogen-fixing strains of corn and wheat. And it is important to know how likely it is that recombinant DNA research will lead to techniques for effectively treating or preventing various types of cancer. Yet there is no experiment we can perform nor any data we can gather that will enable us to *empirically* estimate these probabilities. Nor are these the most problematic probabilities we may want to know. A possibility that weighs heavily on the minds of many who are worried about recombinant DNA research is that this research may lead to negative consequences for human health or for the environment *which have not yet even been thought of*. The history of technology during the last half-century surely demonstrates that this is not a quixotic concern. Yet here again there would appear to be no data we can gather that would help much in estimating the probability of such potential outcomes.

It should be stressed that the problems just sketched are not to be traced simply to a paucity of data. Rather, they are conceptual problems; it is doubtful whether there is *any clear empirical sense* to be made of objective probability assignments to contingencies like those we are considering.

Theorists in the Bayesian tradition may be unmoved by the difficulties we have noted. On their view all probability claims are reports of subjective probabilities.[5] And, a Bayesian might quite properly note, there is no special problem about assigning *subjective* probabilities to

5. For an elaboration of the Bayesian position, see Leonard J. Savage, *The Foundations of Statistics* (New York: John Wiley & Sons, 1954); also cf. Leonard J. Savage, "The Shifting Foundations of Statistics," in Robert G. Colodny, ed., *Logic, Laws and Life* (Pittsburgh: University of Pittsburgh Press, 1977).

outcomes such as those that worried us. But even for the radical Bayesian, there remains the problem of *whose* subjective probabilities ought to be employed in making a *social* or *political* decision. The problem is a pressing one since the subjective probabilities assigned to potential dangers and benefits of recombinant DNA research would appear to vary considerably even among reasonably well informed members of the scientific community.

The difficulties we have been surveying are serious ones. Some might feel they are so serious that they render rational assessment of the risks and benefits of recombinant DNA research all but impossible. I am inclined to be rather more optimistic, however. Almost all of the perils posed by recombinant DNA research require the occurrence of a sequence of separate events. For a chimerical bacterial strain created in a recombinant DNA experiment to cause a serious epidemic, for example, at least the following events must occur:

(1) a pathogenic bacterium must be synthesized
(2) the chimerical bacteria must escape from the laboratory
(3) the strain must be viable in nature
(4) the strain must compete successfully with other micro-organisms which are themselves the product of intense natural selection.[6]

Since *all* of these must occur, the probability of the potential epidemic is the product of the probabilities of each individual contingency. And there are at least two items on the list, namely (2) and (3), whose probabilities are amenable to reasonably straightforward empirical assessment. Thus the product of these two individual probabilities places an upper limit on the probability of the epidemic. For the remaining two probabilities, we must rely on subjective probability assessments of informed scientists. No doubt there will be considerable variability. Yet even here the variability will be limited. In the case of (4), as an example, the available knowledge about microbial natural selection provides no precise way of estimating the probability that a chimerical strain of enfeebled *E. coli* will compete successfully

6. For an elaboration of this point, see Bernard D. Davis, "Evolution, Epidemiology, and Recombinant DNA," in David A. Jackson and Stephen P. Stich, eds., *The Recombinant DNA Debate* (Englewood Cliffs, N.J.: Prentice-Hall, 1979).

outside the laboratory. But no serious scientist would urge that the probability is *high*. We can then use the highest responsible subjective estimate of the probabilities of (1) and (4) in calculating the "worst case" estimate of the risk of epidemic. If in using this highest "worst case" estimate, our assessment yields the result that benefits outweigh risks, then lower estimates of the same probabilities will, of course, yield the same conclusion. Thus it may well be the case that the problems about probabilities we have reviewed will not pose insuperable obstacles to a rational assessment of risks and benefits.

Weighing Harms and Benefits

A second cluster of problems that confronts us in assessing the risks and benefits of recombinant DNA research turns on the assignment of a measure of desirability to the various possible outcomes. Suppose that we have a list of the various harms and benefits that might possibly result from pursuing recombinant DNA research. The list will include such "benefits" as development of an inexpensive way to synthesize human clotting factor and development of a strain of nitrogen-fixing wheat; and such "harms" as release of a new antibiotic-resistant strain of pathogenic bacteria and release of a strain of *E. coli* carrying tumor viruses capable of causing cancer in man.

Plainly, it is possible that pursuing a given policy will result in more than one benefit and in more than one harm. Now if we are to assess the potential impact of various policies or courses of action, we must assign some index of desirability to the possible *total outcomes* of each policy, outcomes which may well include a mix of benefits and harms. To do this we must confront a tangle of normative problems that are as vexing and difficult as any we are likely to face. We must *compare* the moral desirabilities of various harms and benefits. The task is particularly troublesome when the harms and benefits to be compared are of different kinds. Thus, for example, some of the attractive potential benefits of recombinant DNA research are economic: we may learn to recover small amounts of valuable metals in an economically feasible way, or we may be able to synthesize insulin and other drugs inexpensively. By contrast, many of the risks of recombinant DNA research are risks to human life or health. So if we are to take the idea of cost-benefit analysis seriously, we must at some point decide how human lives are to be weighed against economic benefits.

There are those who contend that the need to make such decisions indicates the moral bankruptcy of attempting to employ risk-benefit analyses when human lives are at stake. On the critics' view, we cannot reckon the possible loss of a human life as just another negative outcome, albeit a grave and heavily weighted one. To do so, it is urged, is morally repugnant and reflects a callous lack of respect for the sacredness of human life.

On my view, this sort of critique of the very idea of using risk-benefit analyses is ultimately untenable. It is simply a fact about the human condition, lamentable as it is inescapable, that in many human activities we run the risk of inadvertently causing the death of a human being. We run such a risk each time we drive a car, allow a dam to be built, or allow a plane to take off. Moreover, in making social and individual decisions, we cannot escape weighing economic consequences against the risk to human life. A building code in the Midwest will typically mandate fewer precautions against earthquakes than a building code in certain parts of California. Yet earthquakes are not impossible in the Midwest. If we elect not to require precautions, then surely a major reason must be that it would simply be too expensive. In this judgment, as in countless others, there is no escaping the need to balance economic costs against possible loss of life. To deny that we must and do balance economic costs against risks to human life is to assume the posture of a moral ostrich.

I have been urging the point that it is not *morally objectionable* to try to balance economic concerns against risks to human life. But if such judgments are unobjectionable, indeed necessary, they also surely are among the most difficult any of us has to face. It is hard to imagine a morally sensitive person not feeling extremely uncomfortable when confronted with the need to put a dollar value on human lives. It might be thought that the moral dilemmas engendered by the need to balance such radically different costs and benefits pose insuperable practical obstacles for a rational resolution of the recombinant DNA debate. But here, as in the case of problems with probabilities, I am more sanguine. For while some of the risks and potential benefits of recombinant DNA research are all but morally incommensurable, the most salient risks and benefits are easier to compare. The major risks, as we have noted, are to human life and health. However, the major potential benefits are *also* to human life and health. The potential economic benefits of recombinant DNA research pale in significance when set against the potential for major breakthroughs in our understanding and ability to treat a broad range of conditions, from birth defects to cancer. Those of us, and I confess I am among them, who despair of deciding how lives and economic benefits are to be compared can nonetheless hope to settle our views about recombinant DNA research by comparing the potential risks to life and health with the potential benefits to life and health. Here we are comparing plainly commensurable outcomes. If the balance turns out to be favorable, then we need not worry about factoring in potential economic benefits.

There is a certain irony in the fact that we may well be able to ignore economic factors entirely in coming to a decision about recombinant DNA research. For I suspect that a good deal of the apprehension about recombinant DNA research on the part of the public at large is rooted in the fear that (once again) economic benefits will be weighed much too heavily and potential damage to health and the environment will be weighed much too lightly. The fear is hardly an irrational one. In case after well-publicized case, we have seen the squalid consequences of decisions in which private or corporate gain took precedence over clear and serious threats to health and to the environment. It is the profit motive that led a giant chemical firm to conceal the deadly consequences of the chemical which now threatens to poison the James River and perhaps all of Chesapeake Bay. For the same reason, the citizens of Duluth drank water laced with a known carcinogen. And the ozone layer that protects us all was eroded while regulatory agencies and legislators fussed over the loss of profits in the spray deodorant industry. Yet while public opinion about recombinant DNA research is colored by a growing awareness of these incidents and dozens of others, the case of recombinant DNA is fundamentally different in a crucial respect. The important projected benefits which must be set against the risks of recombinant DNA research are not economic at all, they are medical and environmental.

Problems about Principles

The third problem I want to consider focuses on the following question. Once we have assessed the potential harms and benefits of recombinant DNA research, how should we use this information in coming to a decision? It might be thought that the answer is trivially obvious. To assess the harms and benefits is, after all, just to compute, for each of the various policies that we are considering, what might be called its *expected utility*. The expected utility of a given policy is found by first multiplying the desirability of each possible total outcome by the probability that the policy in question will lead to that total outcome, and then adding the numbers obtained. As we have seen, finding the needed probabilities and assigning the required desirabilities will not be easy. But once we know the expected utility of each policy, is it not obvious that we should choose the policy with the highest expected utility? The answer, unfortunately, is no, it is not at all obvious.

Let us call the principle that we should adopt the policy with the highest expected utility the *utilitarian principle*. The following example should make it clear that, far from being trivial or tautological, the utilitarian principle is a substantive and controversial moral principle. Suppose that the decision which confronts us is whether or not to adopt policy *A*. What is more, suppose we know there is a probability close to 1 that 100,000 lives will be saved if we adopt *A*. However, we also know that there is a probability close to 1 that 1,000 will die as a direct result of our adopting policy *A*, and these people would survive if we did not adopt *A*. Finally, suppose that the other possible consequences of adopting *A* are relatively inconsequential and can be ignored. (For concreteness, we might take *A* to be the establishment of a mass vaccination program, using a relatively risky vaccine.) Now plainly if we take the moral desirability of saving a life to be exactly offset by the moral undesirability of causing a death, then the utilitarian principle dictates that we adopt policy *A*. But many people feel uncomfortable with this result, the discomfort increasing with the number of deaths that would result from *A*. If, to change the example, the choice that confronts us is saving 100,000 lives while causing the deaths of 50,000 others, a significant number of people are inclined to think that the morally right thing to do is to refrain from doing *A*, and "let nature take its course."

If we reject policy *A*, the likely reason is that we also reject the utilitarian principle. Perhaps the most plausible reason for rejecting the utilitarian principle is the view that our obligation to *avoid doing harm* is stronger than our obligation to do good. There are many examples, some considerably more compelling than the one we have been discussing, which seem to illustrate that in a broad range of cases we do feel that our obligation to avoid doing harm is greater than our obligation to do good.[7] Suppose, to take but one example, that my neighbor requests my help in paying off his gambling debts. He owes $5,000 to a certain bookmaker with underworld connections. Unless the neighbor pays the debt immediately, he will be shot. Here, I think we are all inclined to say, I have no strong obligation to give my neighbor the money he needs, and if I were to do so it would be a supererogatory gesture. By contrast, suppose a representative of my neighbor's bookmaker approaches me and requests that I shoot my neighbor. If I refuse, he will see to it that my new car, which cost $5,000, will be destroyed by a bomb while it sits unattended at the curb. In this case, surely, I have a strong obligation not to harm my neighbor, although not shooting him will cost me $5,000.

Suppose that this example and others convince us that we cannot adopt the utilitarian principle, at least not in its most general form, where it purports to be applicable to all moral decisions. What are the alternatives? One cluster of alternative principles would urge that in some or all cases we weigh the harm a contemplated action will cause more heavily than we weigh the good it will do. The extreme form of such a principle would dictate that we ignore the benefits entirely and opt for the action or policy that produces the *least* expected harm. (It is this principle, or a close relation, which emerged in the second reading of the "natural barriers" argument discussed in the third part of Sec-

7. For an interesting discussion of these cases, see J. O. Urmson, "Saints and Heros," in A. I. Melden, ed., *Essays In Moral Philosophy* (Seattle: University of Washington Press, 1958). Also see the discussion of positive and negative duties in Philippa Foot, "The Problem of Abortion and the Doctrine of Double Effect," *Oxford Review* 5 (1967). Reprinted in James Rachels, ed., *Moral Problems* (New York: Harper & Row, 1971).

tion I above.) A more plausible variant would allow us to count both benefits and harms in our deliberations, but would specify how much more heavily harms were to count.

On my view, some moderate version of a "harm-weighted" principle is preferable to the utilitarian principle in a considerable range of cases. *However, the recombinant DNA issue is not one of these cases.* Indeed, when we try to apply a harm-weighted principle to the recombinant DNA case we run head on into a conceptual problem of considerable difficulty. The distinction between doing good and doing harm presupposes a notion of the normal or expectable course of events. Roughly, if my action causes you to be worse off than you would have been in the normal course of events, then I have harmed you; if my action causes you to be better off than in the normal course of events, then I have done you some good; and if my action leaves you just as you would be in the normal course of events, then I have done neither. In many cases, the normal course of events is intuitively quite obvious. Thus in the case of the neighbor and the bookmaker, in the expected course of events I would neither shoot my neighbor nor give him $5,000 to pay off his debts. Thus I am doing good if I give him the money and I am doing harm if I shoot him. But in other cases, including the recombinant DNA case, it is not at all obvious what constitutes the "expected course of events," and thus it is not at all obvious what to count as a harm. To see this, suppose that as a matter of fact many more deaths and illnesses will be prevented as a result of pursuing recombinant DNA research than will be caused by pursuing it. But suppose that there *will* be at least some people who become ill or die as a result of recombinant DNA research being pursued. If these are the facts, then who would be harmed by imposing a ban on recombinant DNA research? That depends on what we take to be the "normal course of events." Presumably, if we do not impose a ban, then the research will continue and the lives will be saved. If this is the normal course of events, then if we impose a ban we have *harmed* those people who would be saved. But it is equally natural to take as the normal course of events the situation in which recombinant DNA research is not pursued. And if *that* is the normal course of events, then those who would have been saved are not harmed by a ban, for they are no worse off than they would be in the normal course of events. However, on this reading of "the normal course of events," if we *fail* to impose a ban, then we have harmed those people who will ultimately become ill or die as a result of recombinant DNA research, since as a result of not imposing a ban they are worse off than they would have been in the normal course of events. I conclude that, in the absence of a theory detailing how we are to recognize the normal course of events, harm-weighted principles have no clear application to the case of recombinant DNA research.

Harm-weighted principles are not the only alternatives to the utilitarian principle. There is another cluster of alternatives that take off in quite a different direction. These principles urge that in deciding which policy to pursue there is a strong presumption in favor of policies that adhere to certain formal moral principles (that is, principles which do not deal with the *consequences* of our policies). Thus, to take the example most directly relevant to the recombinant DNA case, it might be urged that there is a strong presumption in favor of a policy which preserves freedom of scientific inquiry. In its extreme form, this principle would protect freedom of inquiry *no matter what the consequences*; and as we saw in the first part of Section I, this extreme position is exceptionally implausible. A much more plausible principle would urge that freedom of inquiry be protected until the balance of negative over positive consequences reaches a certain specified amount, at which point we would revert to the utilitarian principle. On such a view, if the expected utility of banning recombinant DNA research is a bit higher than the expected utility of allowing it to continue, then we would nonetheless allow it to continue. But if the expected utility of a ban is enormously higher than the expected utility of continuation, banning is the policy to be preferred.[8]

III. Long Term Risks

Thus far in our discussion of risks and benefits, the risks that have occupied us have been what might be termed "short-term" risks, such as the release of a new pathogen. The negative effects of these

8. Carl Cohen defends this sort of limited protection of the formal free inquiry principle over a straight application of the utilitarian principle in his interesting essay, "When May Research Be Stopped?" *New England Journal of Medicine* 296 (1977), reprinted in *The Recombinant DNA Debate*.

events, though they might be long-lasting indeed, would be upon us relatively quickly. However, some of those who are concerned about recombinant DNA research think there are longer-term dangers that are at least as worrisome. The dangers they have in mind stem not from the accidental release of harmful substances in the course of recombinant DNA research, but rather from the unwise use of the *knowledge* we will likely gain in pursuing the research. The scenarios most often proposed are nightmarish variations on the theme of human genetic engineering. With the knowledge we acquire, it is conjectured, some future tyrant may have people built to order, perhaps creating a whole class of people who willingly and cheaply do the society's dirty or dangerous work, as in Huxley's *Brave New World*. Though the proposed scenarios clearly are science fiction, they are not to be lightly dismissed. For if the technology they conjure is not demonstrably achievable, neither is it demonstrably impossible. And if only a bit of the science fiction turns to fact, the dangers could be beyond reckoning.

Granting that potential misuse of the knowledge gained in recombinant DNA research is a legitimate topic of concern, how ought we to guard ourselves against this misuse? One common proposal is to try to prevent the acquisition of such knowledge by banning or curtailing recombinant DNA research now. Let us cast this proposal in the form of an explicit moral argument. The conclusion is that recombinant DNA research should be curtailed, and the reason given for the conclusion is that such research could possibly produce knowledge which might be misused with disastrous consequences. To complete the argument we need a moral principle, and the one which seems to be needed is something such as this:

If a line of research can lead to the discovery of knowledge which might be disastrously misused, then that line of research should be curtailed.

Once it has been made explicit, I think relatively few people would be willing to endorse this principle. For recombinant DNA research is hardly alone in potentially leading to knowledge that might be disastrously abused. Indeed, it is hard to think of an area of scientific research that could *not* lead to the discovery of potentially dangerous knowledge. So if the principle is accepted it would entail that almost all scientific research should be curtailed or abandoned.

It might be thought that we could avoid the extreme consequences just cited by retreating to a more moderate moral principle. The moderate principle would urge only that we should curtail those areas of research where the probability of producing dangerous knowledge is comparatively high. Unfortunately, this more moderate principle is of little help in avoiding the unwelcome consequences of the stronger principle. The problem is that the history of science is simply too unpredictable to enable us to say with any assurance which lines of research will produce which sorts of knowledge or technology. There is a convenient illustration of the point in the recent history of molecular genetics. The idea of recombining DNA molecules is one which has been around for some time. However, early efforts proved unsuccessful. As it happened, the crucial step in making recombinant DNA technology possible was provided by research on restriction enzymes, research that was undertaken with no thought of recombinant DNA technology. Indeed, until it was realized that restriction enzymes provided the key to recombining DNA molecules, the research on restriction enzymes was regarded as a rather unexciting (and certainly uncontroversial) scientific backwater.[9] In an entirely analogous way, crucial pieces of information that may one day enable us to manipulate the human genome may come from just about any branch of molecular biology. To guard against the discovery of that knowledge we should have to curtail not only recombinant DNA research but all of molecular biology.

Before concluding, we would do well to note that there is a profound pessimism reflected in the attitude of those who would stop recombinant DNA research because it might lead to knowledge that could be abused. It is, after all, granted on all sides that the knowledge resulting from recombinant DNA research will have both good and evil potential uses. So it would seem the sensible strategy would be to try to prevent the improper uses of this knowledge rather than trying to prevent the knowledge from ever being uncovered. Those who

9. I am indebted to Prof. Ethel Jackson for both the argument and the illustration.

would take the more extreme step of trying to stop the knowledge from being uncovered presumably feel that its improper use is all but inevitable, that our political and social institutions are incapable of preventing morally abhorrent applications of the knowledge while encouraging beneficial applications. On my view, this pessimism is unwarranted; indeed, it is all but inconsistent. The historical record gives us no reason to believe that what is technologically possible will be done, no matter what the moral price. Indeed, in the area of human genetic manipulation, the record points in quite the *opposite* direction. We have long known that the same techniques that work so successfully in animal breeding can be applied to humans as well. Yet there is no evidence of a "technological imperative" impelling our society to breed people as we breed dairy cattle, simply because we know that it can be done. Finally, it is odd that those who express no confidence in the ability of our institutions to forestall such monstrous applications of technology are not equally pessimistic about the ability of the same institutions to impose an effective ban on the uncovering of dangerous knowledge. If our institutions are incapable of restraining the application of technology when those applications would be plainly morally abhorrent, one would think they would be even more impotent in attempting to restrain a line of research which promises major gains in human welfare.

This essay is an abridged and somewhat modified version of my essay, "The Recombinant DNA Debate: Some Philosophical Considerations," which will appear in *The Recombinant DNA Debate* edited by David A. Jackson and Stephen P. Stich (Englewood Cliffs, N.J.: Prentice-Hall, 1979). I am grateful to the Editors of *Philosophy & Public Affairs* for their detailed and useful suggestions on modifying the essay to make it appropriate for use in this journal.

JAMES L. MUYSKENS   An Alternative Policy for
Obtaining Cadaver Organs
for Transplantation

Two moral principles have been basic to the legal decisions concerning the rights and duties toward the newly dead. They are the duty
to give decent burial and the denial to anyone of a right to ownership
of the dead body for commercial profit (for example, a body cannot be
sold as security for the payment of a debt).[1] The next-of-kin—rather
than the church (as was the case earlier in the West) or the state—
have come to bear the primary responsibility for providing decent
burial.

The familial duty to give decent burial has come to be understood
as a legal right to determine what is to be done to the body in the
interval between death and burial.

> The courts decided that the next-of-kin had a right to receive pos-
> session of the body immediately after death and in the same condi-
> tion it was in at the time of death. This right to possession is based
> upon the principle that each person should have a decent burial
> and it should be the legal duty of his next-of-kin to provide such.[2]

Armed with this right, the family has had the power to deny permission for the use of an organ for transplantation or for the performance
of an autopsy. Significantly, however, in certain cases of criminal
investigation or the settlement of an insurance contract, an autopsy

1. Paul Ramsey, *The Patient as Person* (New Haven: Yale University Press,
1970), pp. 204-205.
2. David Sanders and Jesse Dukeminier, Jr., "Medical Advance and Legal
Lag: Hemodialysis and Kidney Transplant," *U.C.L.A. Law Review* 15, no. 2
(February 1968): 402.

may be performed on the ground that the interest of society takes precedence over the contrary wishes of the family.

In addition to the interests of society and of the family are the wishes of the deceased (for example, his expressed wish that his body be donated to science or that his body not be cremated). The courts have maintained both that the expressed wish of the deceased ought to be carried out and also that the sentiments of the living should be protected. In cases in which the interests of the living and the wishes of the deceased are in conflict, it has not been clear (until recently) how the courts would exercise their "benevolent discretion."[3]

One of the major aims of the Uniform Anatomical Gift Act proposed in 1968 was to guarantee that the wishes of the deceased—in cases in which she or he has expressed a desire to donate organs for transplantation or to bequeath her or his body to medical authorities for their use—not be revoked by next-of-kin. That is, it was proposed that in cases of conflict, the expressed wishes of the deceased take priority over those of the next-of-kin. However, in cases in which the deceased did not express a desire to donate or have known objections to such donations, the next-of-kin may do so. The basic provisions of the Uniform Anatomical Gift Act are:

1. Any individual over eighteen may give all or part of his body for educational, research, therapeutic, or transplantation purposes.

2. If the individual has not made a donation before his death, his next of kin can make it unless there was a known objection by the deceased.

3. If the individual has made such a gift it cannot be revoked by the relatives.

4. If there is more than one person of the same degree of kinship the gift from relatives shall not be accepted if there is known objection by one of them.

5. The gift can be authorized by a card carried by the individual or by written or recorded verbal communication from a relative.[4]

3. Sanders and Dukeminier, "Medical Advance and Legal Lag," p. 399.
4. Robert Veatch, *Death, Dying, and the Biological Revolution* (New Haven: Yale University Press, 1976), p. 269.

All fifty states have adopted the provisions of the Uniform Anatomical Gift Act. Hence, in the United States any individual eighteen years of age or over or, "in the absence of actual notice of contrary indications by the decedent," a member of the decedent's family may give all or any part of the decedent's body for purposes of medical or dental education, research, or transplantation.

Despite this unprecedented legislative action bringing about uniformity in law in all fifty states and providing a relatively simple means for obtaining cadaver organs for transplantation, the great need for suitable donors remains. There is no question that patients die who would not have to die if there was not a shortage of donors.

> It is tragic that, in the United States alone, perhaps 8,000 of the more than 50,000 who die of kidney failure each year, could be helped with a transplant. We have the way but seem to lack the will to save the lives of thousands of human beings each year, either with transplants or hemodialysis.[5]

One would be inclined to suspect that disapproval on the part of the public may account for the severe shortage. However, according to a Gallup Poll published in the *New York Times* (17 January 1968) 70 per cent of adults in the United States approved the donation of their organs after death. As Gerald Leach says, "If willingness to donate were all, there should be no problems with spare hearts, lungs, livers and kidneys from the dead."[6] Unfortunately only a small percentage of those approving of organ transplants have taken the steps to make their own available in the event that they become suitable donors. Further, the pool of potential donors must be vast in order to meet the need, since "only the very rare death provides organs suitable for donation."[7]

Both the cause of death and the circumstance of death are crucial to the suitability of organs for transplantation. The best donors are young persons who die of certain types of injuries: automobile accidents or violence, brain tumors, strokes, cerebral hemorrhage, and

---

5. Veatch, p. 251.
6. Gerald Leach, *The Biocrats* (New York: McGraw Hill, 1970), p. 266.
7. Veatch, p. 270.

other central nervous system lesions. The organs of those who die at an old age or die of cancer, of infection, or of chronic vascular diseases are not suitable for transplantation. Because of damage to the organs, persons who are dead on arrival at the hospital are usually unsuitable donors. In other situations, the time is too short to obtain the required permission or a transplant team is not available at the place of death.

Since one of the fundamental objectives of medical practice is to save lives, and since many more lives could be saved if there were more organs available for transplantation, it is apparent that we should attempt to find a way to secure greater quantities of suitable cadaver organs.

The task of developing an acceptable policy on this matter is difficult because we cannot focus on the need to save lives while ignoring other compelling considerations. In trying to achieve the unquestionably worthy goal of saving lives, one must not violate fundamental duties (for example, a doctor's duty to provide the best care he can for the dying patient in his care) or endanger or diminish other important objectives of society (for example, the preservation of religious freedom and enhancement of respect for life). Certain moral constraints and moral objectives must be considered in devising social policy for securing cadaver organs. Before considering these, let us examine the types of policy possible and some actual policy proposals.

Policies for obtaining cadaver organs can be divided into the general categories of "giving," "taking," "trading," "selling."

(1) Giving of cadaver organs. A number of variations are possible. For example, organs may be
   (a) given by the family of the deceased in response to a request for certain organs;
   (b) given by the deceased prior to imminent death in response to a general appeal for suitable organs.

(2) Routine salvaging of cadaver organs. For example,
   (a) routine removal of any and all useful organs;
   (b) routine removal of certain useful organs.

(3) Trading of cadaver organs. For example, an exchange of credits for organs similar to the blood-bank system.

(4) Selling of suitable cadaver organs.

Of these four categories, the last clearly violates the centuries-old principle that no one is entitled to claim ownership of a dead body for commercial profit. I am not aware of any serious advocates of such a claim, and therefore I shall not discuss it further.

The category of "taking" has obvious advantages when it comes to obtaining the organs necessary for saving lives. Few would argue against the efficiency of "taking" organs. But such a practice could violate certain moral constraints or duties, could endanger values which must be preserved, and could undermine important social objectives.

Jesse Dukeminier and David Sanders have presented a proposal for routine salvaging of cadaver organs. They recommend that law and practice be modified so that

(1) removal of useful cadaver organs is routine practice, leaving them to putrefy is unusual

(2) removal of organs is performed under conditions that do not burden the bereaved persons with the problem

(3) the donor may object during life to removal of his own organs after death, which objection is controlling. If, however, the donor expressly agrees to the use of his organs after death, his next-of-kin has no power of veto

(4) if the donor neither objects nor expressly assents, his next-of-kin may object to removal any time before the organs are removed, which objection is controlling.[8]

Dukeminier and Sanders argue that their proposal satisfies the "first and most important principle of medical ethics" which "is to save life."[9] It allows for persons who have objections to these procedures to

8. Sanders and Dukeminier, "Medical Advance and Legal Lag," p. 410.
9. David Sanders and Jesse Dukeminier, Jr., "Organ Transplantation: A Proposal for Routine Salvaging of Cadaver Organs," *The New England Journal of Medicine* 279, no. 8 (August 1968): 419.

exempt themselves. Hence, they do not see their policy as one that threatens individual autonomy or basic freedoms, such as freedom of religion.

Paul Ramsey and Robert Veatch both argue that policies of "taking" should be rejected. Ramsey offers two major objections to policies of "taking" or routine salvaging.

> . . . The wish to exercise a more ancient wisdom concerning the body ought not to be specially burdened. Jewish people or Jehovah's Witnesses or anyone else holding religious objections, or persons without religious philosophy having deeply felt opinions in this matter, should not have, in hours of grief and suffering, to protrude these objections against the whole edifice of a hospital practice which routinely goes on without their wills.

> A society will be a better human community in which giving and receiving is the rule, not taking for the sake of good to come. . . . The positive consent called for by Gift Acts, answering the need for gifts by encouraging real givers, meets the measure of authentic community among men. The routine taking of organs would deprive individuals of the exercise of the virtue of generosity.[10]

Robert Veatch, who favors a policy of "giving" such as that outlined in the Uniform Anatomical Gift Act, says:

> The strongest objection to proposals for routine salvaging is really one of human values. Do we want a society which conceives of body parts as essentially property of the state to be taken by eminent domain or is that a dangerous misordering of moral priorities? If the state can assume that human bodies are its for the taking (unless contested by the individuals or relatives as in the Dukeminier and Sanders proposal), what will be the implications for less ultimate, less sacred possessions? If the body is essential to the individual's identity, in a society which values personal integrity and freedom, it must be the individual's first of all to control, not only over a lifetime, but within reasonable limits after that life is gone

10. Ramsey, p. 210.

as well. If the body is to be made available to others for personal or societal research, it must be a gift.[11]

But Ramsey objects to the Uniform Anatomical Gift Act as well as to the Dukeminier and Sanders proposal.

> That the kin ought always to obey the decedent's premortem rational will contrary to the respect they actually find it possible to render in disposition of his body remains, for me, a profoundly unpersuasive proposition. . . . Since death is an event that takes place within the company of the family, I would hope that premortem donation of organs will be, so far as possible, familial decisions, as burial is, and not in actual practice individualistic decisions made controlling by law.[12]

He goes on to suggest that the ideal policy would be one of "trading":

> . . . since death is an event in a family, the premortem giving of cadaver organs ought also be if possible a familial or shared decision. So also families that shared in premortem giving of organs could share in freely receiving if one of them needs transplant therapy. This would be—if workable—a civilizing exchange of benefit that is not the same as commerce in organs.[13]

I shall now examine the objections to routine salvaging in order to determine what competing moral values and constraints must be taken into account in devising a morally adequate policy. On the basis of this discussion, I shall suggest a policy that best satisfies these moral demands.

Any routine salvaging policy removes the need to obtain premortem consent from the donor or postmortem consent from the family. Clearly, as Ramsey states, such policies place the burden of action on those who, for whatever reason, object to the removal of organs for transplantation. Contrary to the other types of policy, inaction on the part of the donor or the family is not a sufficient condition for nonparticipation.

I suspect that most people would reject a policy which failed to

---

11. Veatch, pp. 268-269.   12. Ramsey, p. 208.
13. Ramsey, pp. 212-213.

allow for nonparticipation by anyone who wishes not to participate. One ought not to be *compelled* to assist another in this way. Although we have a duty not to harm another, it is not so clear that anyone has a duty to help others when the help entails the postmortem surrender of a part of the body. Further, since some religious groups (for example, Jehovah's Witnesses and Orthodox Jews) forbid the removal of organs from the body, compelling participation would be a denial of religious freedom. An adequate social policy would not infringe on these basic rights. Hence, any routine salvaging policy must allow for nonparticipation.

If a routine salvaging policy is adopted, hospitals should be required to take cognizance of the objections of religious as well as non-religious groups opposed to transplantation so that, for anyone who belonged to such a group, salvaging of organs would not be routine. Thus if a patient states that he is, for example, a "Jehovah's Witness" or a member of the "Society for Burial of Intact Bodies," it would be understood that he is a nonparticipant. Such considerations for non-participation would sufficiently safeguard the rights of self-determin-ism and religious freedom. A policy ought to make it possible for one to exercise his freedom. But it is not necessary to remove all need for effort or initiative in exercising these rights. An appropriate analogy is the selective service system with its provisions for conscientious objection.

Ramsey expresses his concern for the individual having to face the "whole edifice of a hospital practice" if routine salvaging were the operational policy. But this is as much a problem for an effective "giving" policy. To meet the important need for organs to any adequate degree, we would need a more aggressive "giving" policy than we now have. That is, we would need a system of "giving" in which it was expected that most or many would give, or in which hospital officials approached next-of-kin in almost every suitable case to request a do-nation. Such a policy, no less than one of "taking," would be open to Ramsey's objection. In either case, when a clear prior statement has been made by the donor the issue of the individual standing up to the "whole edifice of a hospital practice" does not arise. When the wishes of the donor are not clear, the potential for conflict between next-of-kin and hospital is equally strong in both "taking" and "giving" policies.

A "giving" policy has the disadvantage of requiring family approval at the time of death. The family in its most intense moment of grief must sign or refuse to sign approval forms. Any policy that places the onus of approval on the family at the moment of death is not only insensitive but doomed to failure. When a young person (to take as an example a prime candidate for organ transplantation) suddenly and unexpectedly dies, his family may be dumbfounded, may find it difficult if not impossible to believe that he has died, and yet at the same time be agonizingly aware of the fact that he has died. In addition to being stunned, a family member in grief often bears a sense of guilt. When the family is in such a frame of mind, it would be inclined to see the granting of permission for the removal of any organ from the deceased as hurting or violating or demeaning the loved one.

When we find ourselves in these "boundary situations"—when our lives have become unraveled—we need ritual, routine, and automatic procedures. The procedures ought to be those that reflect our collective judgment expressed in more normal times. (The Gallup Poll referred to earlier is a measure of such a judgment.)

These considerations meet Ramsey's first objection and provide some support for a routine salvaging policy as opposed to policies that rely on consent of next-of-kin at the time of death of the donor.

Ramsey's second major objection to a policy of routine salvaging is that it "would deprive individuals of the exercise of the virtue of generosity." It is certainly true that a routine salvaging policy does not allow for the exercise of generosity with regard to the particular organs routinely salvaged. However, there are other avenues open to anyone for expressing the virtue of generosity.

Of course, as Ramsey says, a society in which "giving and receiving is the rule" will be a better society than one in which good is accomplished only by enforcing policies of "taking." The problem is that experience has demonstrated that the sentiment of benevolence or generosity is not strong enough in a sufficient number of people to operate a society without recourse to rules, regulations, and laws.

Hence, this objection reduces to the obvious truth that society would be better if only we all loved one another.

However, social policies must be designed for the society as it is. Is it responsible to allow some to die on the outside chance that someone will be touched by the spirit of generosity? Is it reasonable to allow those who could be saved to die in order to preserve one of many possible avenues for the expression of generosity? Surely, we would need firmer grounds than this to reject policies of "taking."

Robert Veatch argues that routine salvaging proposals entail that body parts are seen "as essentially property of the state to be taken by eminent domain." He maintains that this is a dangerous precedent. One must always be on guard in protecting the individual from the encroachment of the state. However, as social contract theorists have made clear, not all power vested in the state (the collectivity) is a threat to the individual. The more fundamental question we must ask is whether it is in our self-interest to grant the state the right to lay claim to suitable cadaver organs in all cases in which the individual or his family has not expressly denied the state this right.

This question can be answered by considering what sort of "health insurance" one would choose. What would a rational person be willing to pay (or relinquish) in order to have a chance of relief available (through transplantation) in the event of (say) kidney failure? If it is the case (as it appears to be) that the only way a sufficient number of cadaver kidneys can be made available to all persons in need of them is by adopting some policy of routine salvaging, wouldn't the rational person (setting aside those with religious constraints) be willing to relinquish his right to be buried with his kidneys (should he die and his kidneys are suitable for transplantation) in order to have the protection that the availability of cadaver kidneys provides should he suffer kidney failure? We must ask what a rational person would be willing to pay in order to have the protection the availability of cadaver organs provides. The answer is clear. With regard to organs such as kidneys—given the relatively good chances of successful transplantation—we (pragmatically) ought to be (hence, if acting rationally would be) willing to relinquish our right to be buried intact. Organs which, when transplanted, offer good prospects for relief from a debilitating condition or prevent imminent death, shall be called "life-saving" organs. The case for routine salvaging is being made with regard to the limited class of life-saving organs.

A case for routine salvaging of organs which have not been very successfully transplanted cannot be made on this basis. The potential for saving or prolonging the life of anyone in the "donor" pool should such a person happen to suffer organ failure is extremely small for liver or lung transplants. Such cadaver organs made available now would be a contribution to research which may save lives *later* (perhaps the next generation). In these sorts of cases in which immediate benefit to the individual is extremely remote, the organs (if they are to be obtained at all) should accordingly be obtained by volunteers. It is not in the individual's self-interest to vest power in the state for removal of such organs that would not save or enhance lives. In this area of social policy, a routine practice ought not to be adopted when it cannot be shown to conform to consistent or universal enlightened self-interest. The experimental procedures which require cadaver organs would thus remain as cases for the voluntary exercise of altruism.

It should be noted that unless there is an incredible, unanticipated breakthrough in transplantation technique, only a small percentage of people who die would become actual donors. Hence, it is highly unlikely that a routine salvaging policy would result in our society viewing the body's organs as spare parts, and in that way diminish our respect for the body as an integral part of the person. Because of the unobtrusive way in which a routine salvaging policy can be carried out, it would be less likely to lead to a "spare parts mentality" than an efficient "giving" policy, which would require donor cards or traumatic deathbed decisions.

The most adequate policy will be the one that most completely satisfies the following moral restraints and promotes the following social goals:

(1) Provision of a fitting removal of the body from society.
(2) Protection of the integrity of the corpse.
(3) Protection of the bodily integrity and autonomy of the living.
(4) Saving of lives.

(5) Lack of interference with the attainments of other social objectives.

(6) Assistance for the bereaved survivors.

The following policy of limited routine salvaging optimally meets the criteria of adequacy outlined above:

(1a) Removal of life-saving organs which can be removed without visible damage to the cadaver is routine practice.

(1b) Any individual over eighteen may give all or part of his body for educational, research, therapeutic, or transplantation purposes.

(2) Removal of organs is performed under conditions that do not burden the bereaved persons with the problem.

(3) Permission from the next-of-kin is not required either for removal of life-saving organs or any other uses of the body specified in (1b) for which the individual gave express permission before death. However, the next-of-kin have the right to object to any of these procedures in which case their objection is controlling.

(4) An individual may object during life to removal of his organs after death, which objection is controlling. The burden of action for making this objection known lies with the individual and/or his next-of-kin. Such objection may be made any time before the organs are removed.

(5) The bequest of any individual who wishes to give all or part of his body for purposes stated in (1b) can be authorized by a card carried by the individual or by written or recorded oral communication from a relative.

I am grateful to the Editors of *Philosophy & Public Affairs* for improvements in this essay.

PART III
Medical Paternalism

BERNARD GERT and
CHARLES M. CULVER

Paternalistic Behavior

Discussions of paternalism are often marred by the failure to consider the wide variety of paternalistic acts. Thus Gerald Dworkin in his article "Paternalism" says: "By paternalism I shall understand roughly the interference with a person's liberty of action justified by reasons referring exclusively to the welfare, good, happiness, needs, interests, or values of the person being coerced."[1] All Dworkin's examples are of laws or regulations which he considers paternalistic. Though he does recognize that there is such a thing as "parental paternalism" he simply assumes that it will always involve the parent's attempt "to restrict the child's freedom in various ways" (p. 119). Paternalism in law doubtless does involve interference with liberty most of the time, but this is due to the nature of law, not to the nature of paternalism.[2] The first of the above quotations also suggests that Dworkin incorrectly regards interfering with a person's liberty of action

The material in this paper is the product of a faculty seminar at Dartmouth which included the following members of the Departments of Philosophy, Psychiatry and Religion: Bernard Bergen, Ph.D., K. Danner Clouser, Ph.D. (Department of Humanities, College of Medicine, Hershey Medical Center), Ronald Green, Ph.D., Stanley Rosenberg, Ph.D., Joel Rudinow, Ph.D., Raymond Sobel, M.D., Gary Tucker, M.D., and Peter Whybrow, M.D.

1. In *Morality and the Law*, ed. Richard Wasserstrom (Belmont, CA., 1971), p. 108.

2. Dworkin's view that paternalism always involves the restriction of liberty is the standard one. See, for example, "Criminal Paternalism" by Michael D. Bayles and "Justifications for Paternalism" by Donald H. Regan, both in *The Limits of Law—Nomos XV*, ed. J. Roland Pennock and John W. Chapman (Chicago, 1974), pp. 174–188 and 189–210.

as entailing that the person is being coerced.[3] The following example shows that an adequate account of paternalism must allow not only for paternalistic action in which no person is being coerced but also for paternalistic action which does not involve interfering with anyone's liberty of action.

> Mr. *N*, a member of a religious sect that does not believe in blood transfusions, is involved in a serious automobile accident and loses a large amount of blood. On arriving at the hospital, he is still conscious and informs the doctor of his views on blood transfusion. Immediately thereafter he faints from loss of blood. The doctor believes that if Mr. *N* is not given a transfusion he will die. Thereupon, while Mr. *N* is still unconscious, the doctor arranges for and carries out the blood transfusion. (Similar cases may easily be constructed using antibiotic drugs or vaccines.)

This example shows not only that paternalistic action need not be coercive and need not involve an attempt to interfere with the liberty of action of a person, but also that it need not even involve an attempt to control the behavior of the person. We regard coercive action, which involves the use of threats, as a subclass of attempts to interfere with liberty of action. Attempts at such interference are, in turn, a subclass of attempts to control behavior. Thus, by showing that we can have paternalistic action which does not even involve an attempt to control behavior, we can show that paternalistic action need not be coercive nor involve an attempt to interfere with liberty of action. In the blood transfusion case there was no attempt to control behavior, indeed there was no behavior to control; thus it seems clear that there was no attempt to interfere with liberty of action and no coercive action. The same points can be made by considering an example of paternalistic deception which is intended to affect feelings rather than behavior. Consider a case where a doctor lies to a mother on her deathbed when she asks about her son. The doctor tells her that her son is doing well, although he knows that the son has just been killed trying to escape from prison after having been indicted for multiple rape and murder. The doctor behaved paternalistically but did not attempt to control behavior, to apply coercion, or to interfere with

3. For a fuller account of coercion see *Coercion—Nomos XIV*, ed. J. Roland Pennock and John W. Chapman (Chicago, 1972), especially chaps. 3 and 4.

liberty of action. Even in political rather than personal situations, paternalism may involve deception in order to affect the body rather than behavior—for example, officials surreptitiously introduce fluorides into a city's water supply to reduce tooth decay in the inhabitants.

Of course, many paternalistic acts do involve attempts to control behavior, but even these are not all best described as attempts to deprive a person of freedom.[4] (As shown above, it is clearly wrong to describe all paternalistic acts as involving coercion.) The following is a clear case of paternalism involving the deprivation of freedom.

> Mr. *K* is pacing back and forth on the roof of his five-story tenement and appears to be on the verge of jumping off. When questioned by the police he sounds confused. When interviewed by Dr. *T* in the emergency room, Mr. *K* admits to being afraid that he might jump off the roof and says that he fears he is losing his mind. However, he adamantly refuses hospitalization. Dr. *T* decides that for his own protection, Mr. *K* must be committed to the hospital for a period of forty-eight hours.

The following case, though it might be described as deprivation of freedom, seems more accurately described as depriving a person of opportunity.

> Professor *B* tells his wife that he has had a brief affair with her best friend. On hearing this, his wife becomes very depressed and says that she wants to kill herself. In fact, she once took an overdose of sleeping pills when she was depressed. Before leaving for a class that will be over in two hours he, without telling her, removes all the sleeping pills from the house.[5]

4. Dworkin makes no distinction between "interfering with liberty" and "restricting freedom." There may be no distinction to be made here, but we think it is useful to distinguish between the different ways that one can attempt to control another's behavior. We shall use "depriving of freedom" as the one corresponding most closely to Dworkin's phrases, and distinguish it from other ways of controlling behavior, for example, disabling a person.

5. In this example, whether we regard Professor *B*'s act as paternalistic or not depends upon whether we regard him as depriving his wife of the opportunity to take the sleeping pills. Similar problems arise with regard to companies that are called paternalistic. Suppose a company puts a significantly larger percentage of money per employee into pensions and benefits than most companies do, and a correspondingly smaller one into salaries and wages. Whether we regard the company as paternalistic will depend on whether we regard the company as

There are other paternalistic acts that are best described as disabling. This can involve physically disabling a person; for example, a mother, convinced that her son will be killed if he joins the Marines, breaks his arm in order to prevent him from doing so. This somewhat unusual case may broadly be described as an attempt at behavior control, but the result is not attained by depriving the son of freedom. Knocking someone out by a blow, as one might do to a friend who seemed about to attack an armed robber, can be a paternalistic act, but it is more plausibly described as temporary disabling than as deprivation of freedom. Disabling the will of a person, that is, doing something that takes away his ability to will to do certain kinds of acts can also be paternalistic. Thus certain kinds of aversive conditioning may result in a lack of the ability to will, and may be done primarily to prevent a patient from carrying out actions which are harmful to himself.

All of the paternalistic acts described above involve doing something which needs moral justification. We believe that an essential feature of paternalistic behavior toward a person is the violation of moral rules (or doing that which will require such violations), for example, the moral rules prohibiting deception, deprivation of freedom or opportunity, or disabling. One can even imagine a paternalistic act which involves breaking the moral rule against killing, for example, killing a person who has developed the symptoms of rabies and thus faces a certain and excruciatingly painful death. Obviously one can also act paternalistically by violating the moral rule prohibiting the causing of pain, either physical pain or mental suffering, if it is done in order to prevent what one believes to be even greater pain or suffering, as the following case shows.

---

depriving its employees of the opportunity to spend their money in the way that they choose. If we think the company is paying a fair wage as well as putting more than is required into the pension fund, then it is not correct to view the company as paternalistic. It is often difficult to determine the difference between depriving someone of something, and simply not providing him with that thing. We make no attempt in this paper to resolve this problem. We do claim that an action is paternalistic only when it deprives someone of an opportunity (or in some other way violates a moral rule). We wish to thank Gerald Dworkin for calling our attention to this problem.

Mrs. *B* will undergo surgery in two or three days for a malignant tumor of her right breast. She has obviously understood her situation intellectually, but her mood has been rather blasé and she appears to be rather inappropriately minimizing the emotional gravity of her situation. Dr. *T*'s experience is that women in Mrs. *B*'s situation who before mastectomy do not experience some grief and at least moderate concern about the physical and cosmetic implications of their operation often have a very severe and depressive post-operative course. Though Mrs. *B* has insisted that she does not wish to talk about the effects of the surgery, Dr. *T* talks with her about such effects prior to surgery in order to facilitate her emotional preparation for her impending loss.

This last example also goes against a common view of medical paternalism. If one is presented with the following question: Which doctor is acting paternalistically, one who confronts a patient with a painful truth, or one who withholds the truth in order to avoid the pain it will cause the patient? most will answer that it is the latter, not the former, who is acting paternalistically. But as the example immediately above makes clear, this need not be the case. Which, if either, doctor is acting paternalistically depends upon whether he will proceed with what he thinks is best for the patient regardless of the patient's expressed wishes on the matter. If the patient wants to be told the truth, no matter what, then to withhold it simply to prevent his suffering the effects of being told is paternalistic. But if the patient says that he does not want to be told the truth—say, about his having terminal cancer—then it is paternalistic of the doctor to cause suffering by forcing the truth on the patient on the grounds that it is better for him to face the painful truth now.

With this background, we offer the following definition of paternalistic behavior:

A is acting paternalistically toward *S* if and only if *A*'s behavior (correctly) indicates that *A believes that*:
   (1) his action is for *S*'s good
   (2) he is qualified to act on *S*'s behalf
   (3) his action involves violating a moral rule (or doing that which will require him to do so) with regard to *S*

(4) he is justified in acting on S's behalf independently of S's past, present, or immediately forthcoming (free, informed) consent

(5) S believes (perhaps falsely) that he (S) generally knows what is for his own good.

From this account of paternalistic action it is easy to derive accounts of paternalistic attitudes, persons, laws, and so on, but we shall not consider these matters here. What we wish to do now is to discuss the various features of our definition. There is no dispute about (1). If A is acting paternalistically toward S, then A must have the good of S, not his own good, as the goal of his action. Further, insofar as A's behavior toward S is paternalistic, it is only S's good, not the good of some third party, which is involved. This is not to deny that actions can be partially paternalistic; they can be intended for the good of S and others, including A. But what makes A's action toward S paternalistic is never the good of anyone other than S himself.

Feature (2) requires more discussion. In most of the cases that we have considered, being qualified to act on S's behalf involves having certain professional qualifications. But though paternalism is often practiced by those with professional qualifications—such as doctors, lawyers, and social workers—paternalism can be practiced by anyone who has qualifications which he believes enable him to see better than S what is for S's good. Clearly we do not want to make it impossible for a father to act paternalistically toward his teenage son. The father believes his age and experience qualify him to act on his son's behalf, even against his son's express desires. An average person may act paternalistically toward someone who is mentally retarded or partially senile, and a sane person may act paternalistically toward someone who is not sane. They can do this because they believe that being average (or sane) makes them better able to judge the good of S than S himself. In the same way, a sober person can act paternalistically toward a drunk because he feels, at least at the time, that he can tell what is for the drunk's good better than the drunk. A general belief in A's knowing what is for the good of S better than S does himself is required for paternalistic action, and explains why a small child usually cannot be said to be acting paternalistically toward his parents even when he satisfies all of the other conditions.

Feature (3) involves an expansion of what is normally said about paternalism, namely that it involves a deprivation of freedom of the person toward whom one is acting paternalistically. We have seen that paternalism need not always involve violating the moral rule prohibiting the deprivation of freedom or opportunity, and that it can involve violating the moral rules against killing, causing pain, disabling, depriving of pleasure, deception, or breaking a promise. Paternalism involving breaking a promise is even discussed by Plato, who advocates not returning a weapon to someone who has gone mad, even though you have promised to do so. But an action is not paternalistic unless the person whom *A* intends to benefit is also the person toward whom *A* breaks a moral rule. For example, suppose that, without telling your younger brother, you beat up the street bully and tell him that you will do it again if he bothers your brother. If this act is paternalistic toward your brother, as we think it is, it is not so because you have broken a moral rule by beating up the bully. It is paternalistic because you have deceived your younger brother by taking an action which normally would require his consent. Thus, acting without his consent counts as deception.

The paternalistic act need not itself constitute a violation of moral rules, it may involve only doing that which will require one to violate a rule. Giving the blood transfusion to the unconscious member of the religious sect is a paternalistic action which does not itself constitute a violation of any moral rule, but which does involve doing that which will require one to violate a moral rule. For, if the person lives, the doctor must either deceive him regarding the blood transfusion or cause him painful feelings by informing him of the action taken. Since the doctor's initial act requires him to violate a moral rule with regard to his patient, we count it as a paternalistic act.

In our opinion, violating a moral rule involves doing something that would be morally wrong unless one has an adequate justification for doing it. Thus, killing, causing pain (mental or physical), disabling, and depriving of freedom, opportunity, or pleasure are all violations of moral rules. The same is true of deceiving, breaking a promise, and cheating. Paternalistic behavior always involves violating one of these rules (or doing that which will require one to do so) with regard to the person you intend to benefit, independently of his past, present, or immediately forthcoming consent. It is customary to view killing, deceiving and breaking a promise as violations of moral rules, but there is no such tradition with regard to causing someone mental or physical pain, or disabling him, although to do so without adequate justification, is clearly immoral. We see no reason for distinguishing killing and deceiving from causing pain and disabling and think it most fruitful to regard all of these acts, as well as depriving of freedom or opportunity, as violations of moral rules.[6]

Feature (4) makes clear that A believes that he has the moral justification for violating a moral rule with regard to S, and that his action on S's behalf does not need S's past, present or immediately forthcoming consent. A may believe this because A thinks that he will at some future time obtain S's retrospective consent. Though belief about future consent may justify A's action, it does not prevent the action from being paternalistic. If A has S's consent to act on S's behalf, or if A expects S's immediately forthcoming consent for A's action, then an action which might otherwise be paternalistic is not so. For example, I pull someone from the path of an oncoming car which I believe he does not see. If I act because I think that immediately upon being apprised of the facts he will approve of my action, my action is

6. For a fuller account of moral rules, including an account of how one can justify a violation of a moral rule see *The Moral Rules*, by Bernard Gert (New York, 2nd paperback ed., 1975). If one prefers the language of rights to that of moral rules, one might plausibly hold that all paternalistic behavior involves the violation of a person's rights. The close connection between rights and liberties may then partly explain the widely held but mistaken view that paternalism always involves the restriction of liberty of action. For example, in the blood transfusion case, it is plausible to say that we are violating the patient's rights, but it is not plausible to say that we are restricting his liberty of action. Similarly, paternalistic behavior involving deception may sometimes be taken as violating the person's right to know, when it cannot be taken as restricting his liberty of action. There may be no substantive difference between violating a moral rule (or doing that which will require one to do so) with regard to someone independently of his past, present, or immediately forthcoming consent, and violating his rights. However, since we find the terminology of moral rules to be clearer than that of rights, we have presented our analysis of paternalism solely in terms of violating a moral rule.

not paternalistic even though it may satisfy all the other conditions of paternalistic behavior. But if I think that he is trying to commit suicide because of a temporary depression and that he will thank me when he recovers, then my act is paternalistic. Of course, there are borderline cases.

Past, present, or immediately forthcoming consent removes *A*'s act from the class of paternalistic acts. For example, suppose a very distraught patient comes to a psychiatrist and says that he knows that he badly needs treatment and that he would like the psychiatrist's advice about whether to be hospitalized. The psychiatrist is not acting paternalistically when he urges the patient to enter the hospital.[7] Then suppose that, later, the patient wishes to be discharged from the hospital and the psychiatrist refuses permission because he thinks the patient may do himself serious harm if he is allowed to leave. The psychiatrist's refusal is a paternalistic act. Future consent, though it may justify *A*'s act, does not make the action nonpaternalistic. But future consent is not the only thing which can justify paternalistic acts: prevention of bad consequences if they are significant enough may also justify them.

Feature (5) is presupposed in many accounts of paternalism, but rarely is made explicit. We can be paternalistic only toward those whom we regard as believing themselves to be capable of acting on their own behalf. Thus we cannot act paternalistically toward infants and animals unless we believe them to have this sort of self-consciousness. There is, of course, an analogue to paternalism in our treatment of some animals, but it simply muddies the conceptual waters to allow for paternalistic action toward animals and infants. One can act paternalistically toward children, especially older children, for we have

---

7. We might call this paternal behavior and distinguish it from paternalistic behavior in that it does not involve violating a moral rule with regard to *S* independently of *S*'s past, present, or immediately forthcoming consent. We do not intend this statement to be taken as a complete account of paternal behavior.

It should be noted that persons can disagree as to whether behavior is paternal or paternalistic (see fn. 5). Also, we recognize that the term "paternalistic" is often used to describe behavior that we think is more appropriately described as paternal, but we think this no more significant to our analysis than the fact that "jealous" is often used to describe an attitude which is more appropriately described as envious is significant for an analysis of jealousy.

no desire to maintain the paradoxical position that a father cannot act paternalistically toward his children. We can act paternalistically toward those who, we believe, do not, in fact, know what is for their own good, but we cannot act paternalistically toward someone whom we do not regard as believing that he knows what is for his own good.[8]

Now that we have given our definition of paternalism and explained it in some detail, let us consider some cases of psychiatric intervention and see whether the account is of any help in determining whether they are paternalistic or not.

Mrs. *P*, on her first visit as an out-patient, is insistent during the last few minutes of her session that Dr. *T* give her some medicine for her nerves and for the vague, poorly localized pains which she describes. He feels there is no medical reason for her to have medication but judges that if he refuses her request outright, a useful and productive initial interview will end on a very sour note. However, he believes strongly in not administering active drugs when there is no medical reason for doing so; therefore, he writes her a prescription for a week's supply of a placebo and makes a note on her chart to discuss the issue of medication with her in detail at their next week's appointment.

Dr. *T*'s act is clearly paternalistic: he has given her a placebo for what he believes is her own good; he believes he is qualified to carry out such an act on her behalf; he knows he is deceiving her, but believes that he is justified in acting independently of her consent (in this case, even of her knowledge); further he views her as obviously being someone who believes she knows what is for her own good (e.g. to be given a drug). Note that he has not restricted her liberty. Nor has he controlled her behavior: he acted paternalistically to prevent her having bad feelings, not to prevent or encourage any actions on her part.

8. Throughout our analysis we assume that *A*'s beliefs are at least plausible, though they need not be true. If *A*'s beliefs are wildly false, for example, he thinks flowers believe they know what is best for them, then we may hesitate to maintain that he is acting paternalistically toward the flowers when he waters them though he believes that they would prefer to remain dry. We are indebted to Timothy Duggan for calling our attention to this point.

Since this is an instance of paternalism, it requires moral justification. In this case Dr. *T* could attempt to justify giving a placebo (thereby breaking the moral rule prohibiting deception) by making several claims. He could claim that this action was preferable to giving her an active drug, an action that would have been contrary to his proper duty as a physician and would have needlessly exposed her to the risks always attendant upon ingesting any active compound. He could also claim that giving her a placebo was better than flatly refusing her a prescription, an act which would have resulted in her mental suffering.

The morality of giving placebos is an issue about which rational persons may and do disagree. On the basis of the information given in the example we agree that giving any active drug would clearly be wrong; nevertheless, there is insufficient reason to believe that the possible mental suffering caused by Dr. *T*'s refusal would, on balance, be adequate to justify his deception of Mrs. *P*.

Dr. *T* is leading a new therapy group during its second session. The group consists of patients who have all claimed to have difficulty in relating to other people.

One patient, Mr. *G*, is a single professional man in his early 30s who has complained of an inability to maintain lasting friendships with either men or women. It has become apparent to Dr. *T* through watching the group interaction that Mr. *G*, while not totally unlikable, has a penchant for being self-centered, critical of others, and smugly certain about his own opinions. It has also become apparent that Mr. *G* has little insight into these characteristics and the way they irritate other members of the group. Dr. *T* believes it would be useful for Mr. *G* to acquire insight into the effect his personal style has on others. Of course, whether Mr. *G* will then try to change his style will be his own decision.

Accordingly, midway through the session, Dr. *T* begins to encourage other group members to confront Mr. *G* with their feelings about him, despite Mr. *G*'s obvious anger and great discomfort when they begin to do so.

This satisfies four of the five elements of the definition: Dr. *T* believes that confrontation is for Mr. *G*'s good, believes that he is qualified to act on Mr. *G*'s behalf, knows that he is violating a moral rule by causing Mr. *G* mental suffering, and thinks that Mr. *G* is someone who believes he knows what is for his own good. What is not clear from the example as given is whether Dr. *T* believes he is justified in urging confrontation independently of Mr. *G*'s consent. This is not clear because nothing is specified about the nature of the prior agreement between Dr. *T* and Mr. *G*; in particular, whether Mr. *G* has or has not consented to confrontation-type activities (i.e. experiencing emotional pain in the hope of achieving greater self-understanding) and, further, whether Dr. *T*'s actions are or are not independent of any consent Mr. *G* has given. Thus we do not know on the information given whether Dr. *T*'s actions are paternalistic. Dr. *T* might claim that Mr. *G*'s presence in group therapy demonstrates implicit consent to being confronted in an emotionally painful way, but that claim would seem weak if Mr. *G* genuinely had no such expectations.

We stress this example because it seems similar to the dilemma posed by many psychiatric interventions: whether they are paternalistic (and thus require justification) turns heavily on the nature and quality of the consent given by the patient and the degree to which the psychiatrist acts independently of that consent for what he feels is the good of the patient.

In this case, if Dr. *T* has obtained consent so that Mr. *G* has agreed to be exposed to emotionally painful experiences then Dr. *T*'s actions are not paternalistic. If consent has not been obtained, then he is acting paternalistically. He could try to justify his actions on the grounds that by causing Mr. *G* to suffer emotionally for a short period now, he might decrease Mr. *G*'s long-term suffering afterward. This might be true and, of course, is the case with many medical interventions. However we believe it would be unwarranted for Dr. *T* to make this decision unilaterally in a setting where Mr. *G* could have easily been allowed to decide ahead of time whether *he* was willing to gamble on the exchange of more emotional pain now for possibly less later. Thus if Mr. *G*'s consent had not been sought, we would view Dr. *T*'s actions as unjustified paternalism.

We think that the account presented here clarifies many of the features of paternalism. It explains why doctors and others usually resist the charge of paternalism. People generally do not want to be in a position where they have to justify their actions. Thus even though our account does not allow paternalism to degenerate into a term of abuse—for there can be justified paternalism—it makes clear that paternalism involves violating a moral rule without consent and thus requires justification. We can also understand why the concept of paternalism is so closely tied to the notion of informed consent. Particularly in the doctor-patient relationship, it is often not clear whether and to what extent the patient has given his consent to the doctor. This vagueness is evident in the example of the patient in group therapy.

In addition to clarifying the concept of paternalism, we think that the description we have provided allows for some interesting empirical research. For example, what factors in medical training lead a doctor to act paternalistically? To what extent would awareness that one was acting paternalistically (as defined in this paper) decrease (or increase) one's tendency to act paternalistically? Is there a significant difference between doctors who often act paternalistically and those who do so infrequently with regard to their belief about whether people generally know what is for their own good?

ALLEN BUCHANAN   Medical Paternalism

I

There is evidence to show that among physicians in this country the
medical paternalist model is a dominant way of conceiving the physician-patient relationship. I contend that the practice of withholding
the truth from the patient or his family, a particular form of medical
paternalism, is not adequately supported by the arguments advanced
to justify it. Beyond the issue of telling patients the truth is the distinction between "ordinary" and "extraordinary" therapeutic measures,
a distinction which, I argue, both expresses and helps to perpetuate
the dominance of the medical paternalist model.

There are two main types of arguments against paternalism. First
are the arguments that rely upon a theory of moral rights rooted in a
conception of personal autonomy. These arguments are more theoretically interesting and perhaps in the end they are the strongest
arguments against paternalism. Second are the arguments that meet
the paternalist on his own ground and then attempt to cut it from
beneath him by showing that his arguments are defective. I shall concentrate on the second type of antipaternalist argument because I
wish my arguments to have some practical effect, and I believe that
this goal can best be achieved if they are directed against paternalist
justifications which are actually employed by the practitioners of
medical paternalism. Further, the arguments I advance require a
minimum of theoretical baggage. The strength of a rights-based attack
on paternalism depends ultimately upon whether a rational founda-

tion for the relevant theory of rights can be produced. It would be unfortunate if successful attacks on medical paternalism had to await the development and defense of a full-blown theory of moral rights. By articulating the inadequacy of the justifications which the paternalist himself advances, however, one need rely only upon those moral views to which the paternalist himself subscribes. My goal, then, is to present effective criticisms of medical paternalist practices which rely upon a minimal base of moral agreement between the paternalist and his critic.

II

Paternalism is usually characterized as interference with a person's liberty of action, where the alleged justification of the interference is that it is for the good of the person whose liberty of action is thus restricted.[1] To focus exclusively on interference with liberty of *action*, however, is to construe paternalism too narrowly. If a government lies to the public or withholds information from it, and if the alleged justification of its policy is that it benefits the public itself, the policy may properly be called paternalistic.

On the one hand, there may be a direct connection between such a policy and actual interference with the citizen's freedom to act. In order to withhold information from the public, agents of the government may physically interfere with the freedom of the press to gather, print, or distribute the news. Or government officials may misinform the public in order to restrict its freedom to perform specific acts. The police, for example, may erect signs bearing the words "Detour: Maintenance Work Ahead" to route unsuspecting motorists around the wreckage of a truck carrying nerve gas. On the other hand, the connection between withholding of information and actual interference with freedom of action may be indirect at best. To interfere with the public's freedom of information the government need not actually interfere with anyone's freedom to act—it may simply not divulge certain information. Withholding information may preclude an *informed* decision, and it may interfere with attempts to reach an in-

1. See, for example, G. Dworkin's paper "Paternalism," in S. Gorovitz et al., *Moral Problems in Medicine* (Englewood Cliffs, NJ; Prentice-Hall, 1976), p. 185.

formed decision, without thereby interfering with a person's freedom
to decide and to act on his decision. Even if I am deprived of information which I must have if I am to make an informed decision, I may
still be free to decide and to act.

Granted the complexity of the relations between information and
action, it seems plausible to expand the usual characterization of
paternalism as follows: paternalism is interference with a person's
freedom of action or freedom of information, or the deliberate dissemination of misinformation, where the alleged justification of interfering or misinforming is that it is for the good of the person who is interfered with or misinformed. The notion of freedom of information is,
of course, unsatisfyingly vague, but the political examples sketched
above along with the medical examples to follow will make it clearer.
We can now turn to a brief consideration of evidence for the claim
that medical paternalism is a widespread phenomenon in our society.

III

The evidence for medical paternalism is both direct and indirect. The
direct evidence consists of the findings of surveys which systemati-
cally report physicians' practices concerning truth-telling and decision-
making and of articles and discussions in which physicians and others
acknowledge or defend paternalistic medical practices. The indirect
evidence is more subtle. One source of indirect evidence for the pervasiveness of medical paternalist attitudes is the language we use to
describe physician-patient interactions. Let us now consider some of
the direct evidence.

Though there are many ways of classifying cases of medical paternalism, two distinctions are especially important. We can distinguish
between the cases in which the patient is legally competent and those
in which the patient is legally incompetent; and between those cases
in which the intended beneficiary of paternalism is the patient himself and those in which the intended beneficiary is the patient's
guardian or one or more members of the patient's family. The first
distinction classifies cases according to the *legal status of the patient*,
the second according to the *object of paternalism*.

A striking revelation of medical paternalism in dealings with legally
competent adults is found in Donald Oken's essay, "What to Tell

Cancer Patients: A Study of Medical Attitudes."[2] The chief conclusion of this study of internists, surgeons, and generalists is that ". . . there is a strong and general tendency to withhold" from the patient the information that he has cancer. Almost 90 percent of the total group surveyed reported that their usual policy is not to tell the patient that he has cancer. Oken also notes that "no one reported a policy of informing every patient." Further, Oken reports that some physicians falsified diagnoses.

> Some physicians avoid even the slightest suggestion of neoplasia and quite specifically substitute another diagnosis. Almost everyone reported resorting to such falsification on at least a few occasions, most notably when the patient was in a far-advanced stage of illness at the time he was seen.[3]

The physicians' justifications for withholding or falsifying diagnostic information were uniformly paternalistic. They assumed that if they told the patient he had cancer they would be depriving him of all hope and that the loss of hope would result in suicidal depression or at least in a serious worsening of the patient's condition.

A recent malpractice case illustrates paternalistic withholding of information of a different sort. As in the Oken study, the object of paternalism was the patient and the patient was a legally competent adult. A bilateral thyroidectomy resulted in permanent paralysis of the patient's vocal cords. The patient's formerly healthy voice became frail and weak. The damage suit was based on the contention that by failing to tell the patient of the known risks to her voice, the physician had violated his duty to obtain informed consent for the operation. The physician's testimony is clearly paternalistic.

> In court the physician was asked "You didn't inform her of any dangers or risks involved? Is that right?" Over his attorney's objections, the physician responded, "Not specifically. . . . I feel that were I to point out all the complications—or even half the complica-

2. In *Moral Problems in Medicine*, p. 112. Oken's study was first published in 1967.
3. Oken, p. 113.

tions—many people would refuse to have anything done, and therefore would be much worse off."[1]

There is also considerable evidence of medical paternalism in the treatment of legally incompetent individuals through the withholding of information from the patients or their guardians or both.[5]

The law maintains that it is the parents who are primarily responsible for decisions concerning the welfare of their minor children.[6] Nonetheless, physicians sometimes assume primary or even total responsibility for the most awesome and morally perplexing decisions affecting the welfare of the child.

The inescapable need to make such decisions arises daily in neonate intensive care units. The most dramatic decisions are whether to initiate or not initiate, or to continue or discontinue life-sustaining therapy. Three broad types of cases are frequently discussed in recent literature. First, there are infants who are in an asphyxiated condition at birth and can be resuscitated but may suffer irreversible brain-damage if they survive. Second, there are infants with Down's syndrome (mongolism) who have potentially fatal but surgically correctable congenital cardiovascular or gastrointestinal defects. Third, there are infants with spina bifida, a congenital condition in which there is an opening in the spine and which may be complicated by paralysis and hydrocephaly. New surgical techniques make it possible to close the spine and drain the fluid from the brain, but a large percentage of the infants thus treated suffer varying degrees of permanent brain-damage and paralysis.

A. Shaw notes that some physicians undertake the responsibility

4. *Malpractice Digest* (St. Paul, MN: The St. Paul Property and Liability Insurance Company, July-August 1977), p. 6.

5. It is interesting to note that according to both the usual and the expanded characterization of paternalism stated above, only a person who has certain physical and mental capacities can be an object of paternalism, since it is only when these capacities are present that it is correct to speak of interfering with that individual's freedom of action, misinforming him, or withholding information from him.

6. For a helpful summary, see J. A. Robertson and N. Frost, "Passive Euthanasia of Defective Newborn Infants: Legal Considerations," *The Journal of Pediatrics* 88, no. 5 (1976): 883-889.

for making decisions about life and death for defective newborns in order to relieve parents of the trauma and guilt of making a decision. He cites the following comment as an example of this position.

> At the end it is usually the doctor who has to decide the issue. It is . . . cruel to ask the parents whether they want their child to live or die. . . .[7]

We have already seen that the information which physicians withhold may be of at least two different sorts. In the cases studied by Oken, physicians withhold the diagnosis of cancer from their patients. In the thyroidectomy malpractice case the physician did not withhold the diagnosis but did withhold information about known risks of an operation. The growing literature on life or death decisions for defective neonates reveals more complex paternalistic practices. Some physicians routinely exclude parents from significant participation in decision-making either by not informing the parents that certain choices can or must be made, or by describing the child's condition and the therapeutic options in such a skeletal way as to preclude genuinely informed consent.

A case cited by Shaw is a clear example of a physician withholding from parents the information that there was a choice to be made.

> Baby A was referred to me at 22 hours of age with a diagnosis of esophageal atresia and tracheoesophageal fistula. The infant, the firstborn of a professional couple in their early thirties had obvious signs of mongolism, about which they were fully informed by the referring physician. After explaining the nature of the surgery to the distraught father, I offered him the operative consent. His pen hesitated briefly above the form and then as he signed, he muttered, "I have no choice, do I?" He didn't seem to expect an answer and I gave him none. The esophageal anomaly was corrected in routine fashion, and the infant was discharged to a state institution for the retarded without ever being seen again by either parent.[8]

7. Shaw, "Dilemmas of 'Informed Consent' in Children," *The New England Journal of Medicine* 289, no. 17 (1973): 886.
8. Shaw, p. 885.

The following description of practices in a neonate intensive care unit at Yale illustrates how parents may be excluded because of inadequate information about the child's condition or the character of various therapeutic options.

> Parents routinely signed permits for operation though rarely had they seen their children's defects or had the nature of various management plans and their respective prognoses clearly explained to them. Some physicians believed that parents were too upset to understand the nature of the problems and the options for care. Since they believed informed consent had no meaning in these circumstances, they either ignored the parents or simply told them that the child needed an operation on the back as the first step in correcting several defects. As a result, parents often felt completely left out while the activities of care proceeded at a brisk pace.[9]

Not every case in which a physician circumvents or overrides parental decision-making is a case of paternalism toward the parents. In ignoring the parents' primary legal responsibility for the child, the physician may not be attempting to shield the parents from the burdens of responsibility—he may simply be attempting to protect what he perceives to be the interests of the child.

These examples are presented, not as conclusive evidence for the claim that paternalist practices of the sorts discussed above are widespread, but as illustrations of the practical relevance of the justifications for medical paternalism, which I shall now articulate and criticize.

IV

In spite of the apparent pervasiveness of paternalistic practices in medicine, no systematic justification of them is available for scrutiny. Nonetheless, there appear to be at least three main arguments which advocates of paternalism could and sometimes do advance in justification of withholding information or misinforming the patient or his

9. R. Duff and A. Campbell, "Moral and Ethical Dilemmas in the Special-Care Nursery," *The New England Journal of Medicine* 289, no. 17 (1973): 893.

family. Since withholding information seems to be more commonly practiced and advocated than outright falsification, I shall consider the three arguments only as justifications of the former rather than the latter. Each of these arguments is sufficiently general to apply to each of the types of cases distinguished above. For convenience we can label these three arguments (A) the Prevention of Harm Argument, (B) the Contractual Version of the Prevention of Harm Argument, and (C) the Argument from the Inability to Understand.

The Prevention of Harm Argument is disarmingly simple. It may be outlined as follows.

1. The physician's duty—to which he is bound by the Oath of Hippocrates—is to prevent or at least to minimize harm to his patient.
2. Giving the patient information X will do great harm to him.
3. (Therefore) It is permissible for the physician to withhold information X from the patient.

Several things should be noted about this argument. First of all, the conclusion is much weaker than one would expect, granted the first premise. The first premise states that it is the physician's *duty* to prevent or minimize harm to the patient, not just that it is *permissible* for him to do so. However, since the weaker conclusion—that withholding information is permissible—seems more intuitively plausible than the stronger one, I shall concentrate on it.

Second, the argument as it stands is invalid. From the claims that (1) the physician's duty (or right) is to prevent or minimize harm and that (2) giving information X will do the patient great harm, it does not follow that (3) it is permissible for the physician to withhold information X from the patient. At least one other premise is needed: (2′) giving information X will do greater harm to the patient on balance than withholding the information will.

The addition of (2′) is no quibble. Once (2′) is made explicit we begin to see the tremendous weight which this paternalist argument places on the physician's powers of judgment. He must not only determine that giving the information will do harm or even that it will do great harm. He must also make a complex comparative judgment. He must judge that withholding the information will result in less harm on balance than divulging it. Yet neither the physicians interviewed by Oken nor those discussed by Shaw even mention this comparative judgment in their justifications of withholding information. They simply state that telling the truth will result in great harm to the patient or his family. No mention was made of the need to compare this expected harm with harm which might result from withholding the information, and no recognition of the difficulties involved in such a comparison was reported.

Consider two of the cases described above: a terminal cancer case and the thyroidectomy case. In order to justify withholding the diagnosis of terminal cancer from the patient the physician must not only determine that informing the patient would do great harm but that the harm would be greater on balance than whatever harm may result from withholding information. Since the notion of "great harm" here is vague unless a context for comparison is supplied, we can concentrate on the physician's evidence for the judgment that the harm of informing is greater on balance than the harm of withholding. Oken's study showed that the evidential basis for such comparative judgments was remarkably slender.

> It was the exception when a physician could report known examples of the unfavorable consequences of an approach which differed from his own. It was more common to get reports of instances in which different approaches has turned out satisfactorily. Most of the instances in which unhappy results were reported to follow a differing policy turned out to be vague accounts from which no reliable inference could be drawn.

Oken then goes on to focus on the nature of the anticipated harm.

> It has been repeatedly asserted that disclosure is followed by fear and despondency which may progress into overt depressive illness or culminate in suicide. This was the opinion of the physicians in the present study. Quite representative was the surgeon who stated, "I would be afraid to tell and have the patient in a room with a window." When it comes to actually documenting the prevalence of such ontoward reactions, it becomes difficult to find reliable evi-

dence. Instances of depression and profound upsets came quickly
to mind when the subject was raised, but no one could report more
than a case or two, or a handful at most. . . . The same doctors
could remember many instances in which the patient was told and
seemed to do well.[10]

It is not simply that these judgments of harm are made on the basis
of extremely scanty evidence. The problem goes much deeper than
that. To say simply that physicians base such judgments on extremely
weak evidence is to overlook three important facts. First, the judgment
that telling the truth would result in suicidal depression is an unqualified *psychiatric* generalization. So even if there were adequate evidence for this generalization or, more plausibly, for some highly
qualified version of it, it is implausible to maintain that ordinary physicians are in a position to recognize and assess the evidence properly
in a given case. Second, it is doubtful that psychiatric specialists are
in possession of any such reliable generalization, even in qualified
form. Third, the paternalist physician is simply assuming that suicide
is not a rational choice for the terminally ill patient.

If we attempt to apply the Prevention of Harm Argument to cases
in which the patient's family or guardian is the object of paternalism,
other difficulties become apparent. Consider cases of withholding information from the parents of a neonate with Down's syndrome or
spina bifida. The most obvious difficulty is that premise (1) states
only that the physician has a duty (or a right) to prevent or minimize
harm to the patient, not to his family. If this argument is to serve as a
justification of paternalism toward the infant patient's family, the
advocate of paternalism must advance and support one or the other of
two quite controversial premises. He must either add premise (1′) or
replace premise (1) with premise (1″):

(1′) If X is a guardian or parent of a patient Y and Y is the patient
      of physician Z, then X is thereby a patient of physician Z as
      well.

(1″) It is the duty of the physician to prevent or minimize harm to
      his patient and to the guardian or family of his patient.

10. Oken, "What to Tell Cancer Patients," pp. 112, 113.

Since both the law and common sense maintain that one does not become a patient simply by being related to a patient, it seems that the best strategy for the medical paternalist is to rely on (1″) rather than on (1′).

Reliance on (1″), however, only weakens the case for medical paternalism toward parents of defective neonates. For now the medical paternalist must show that he has adequate evidence for psychiatric predictions the complexity of which taxes the imagination. He must first determine all the relevant effects of telling the truth, not just on the parents themselves, but on siblings as well, since whatever anguish or guilt the parents will allegedly feel may have significant effects on their other children. Next he must ascertain the ways in which these siblings—both as individuals and as a peer group—will respond to the predicted anguish and guilt of their parents. Then the physician must determine how the siblings will respond to each other. Next he must consider the possible responses of the parents to the responses of the children. And, of course, once he has accomplished all of this, the physician must look at the other side of the question. He must consider the possible harmful effects of withholding information from patients or of preventing them from taking an active part in decision-making. The conscientious paternalist must consider not only the burdens which the exercise of responsibility will allegedly place upon the parents, and indirectly upon their children, but also the burdens of guilt, self-doubt, and shame which may result from the parents' recognition that they have abdicated their responsibility.

In predicting whether telling the truth or withholding information will cause the least harm for the family as a whole, the physician must first make intrapersonal comparisons of harm and benefit for each member of the family, if the information is divulged. Then he must somehow coalesce these various intrapersonal net harm judgments into an estimate of the total net harm which divulging the information will do to the family as a whole. Then he must make similar intrapersonal and interpersonal net harm judgments about the results of not telling the truth. Finally he must compare these totals and determine which course of action will minimize harm to the family as a whole.

Though the problems of achieving defensible predictions of harm

as a basis for paternalism are clearest in the case of defective neonates, they are in no way peculiar to those cases. Consider the case of
a person with terminal cancer. To eliminate the complication of interpersonal net harm comparisons, let us suppose that this person has no
relatives and is himself legally competent. Suppose that the physician
withholds information of the diagnosis because he believes that knowledge of the truth would be more harmful than withholding the truth.
I have already indicated that even if we view this judgment of comparative harm as a purely clinical judgment—more specifically a clinical psychiatric judgment—it is difficult to see how the physician could
be in a position to make it. But it is crucial to note that the notions of
harm and benefit appropriate to these deliberations are not exclusively
clinical notions, whether psychiatric or otherwise. In taking it upon
himself to determine what will be most beneficial or least harmful to
this patient the physician is not simply making ill-founded medical
judgments which someday might be confirmed by psychiatric research. He is making *moral* evaluations of the most basic and problematic kind.

The physician must determine whether it will be better for the
patient to live his remaining days in the knowledge that his days are
few or to live in ignorance of his fate. But again, this is a gross simplification: it assumes that the physician's attempt to deceive the patient
will be successful. E. Kübler-Ross claims that in many, if not most,
cases the terminally ill patient will guess or learn his fate whether the
physician withholds the diagnosis from him or not.[11] Possible harm
resulting from the patient's loss of confidence in the physician or from
a state of uncertainty over his prospects must be taken into account.

Let us set aside this important complication and try to appreciate
what sorts of factors would have to be taken into account in a well-
founded judgment that the remainder of a person's life would be
better for that person if he did not know that he had a terminal illness
than if he did.

Such a judgment would have to be founded on a profound knowledge of the most intimate details of the patient's life history, his characteristic ways of coping with personal crises, his personal and

11. Kübler-Ross, excerpts from *Death and Dying*, quoted in *Moral Problems
in Medicine*, p. 122.

vocational commitments and aspirations, his feelings of obligation toward others, and his attitude toward the completeness or incompleteness of his experience. In a society in which the personal physician was an intimate friend who shared the experience of families under his care, it would be somewhat more plausible to claim that the physician might possess such knowledge. Under the present conditions of highly impersonal specialist medical practice it is quite a different matter.

Yet even if the physician could claim such intimate personal knowledge, this would not suffice. For he must not only predict, but also *evaluate*. On the basis of an intimate knowledge of the patient as a person, he must determine which outcome would be *best* for that person. It is crucial to emphasize that the question which the physician must pose and answer is whether ignorance or knowledge will make possible a life that is better *for the patient himself*. The physician must be careful not to confuse this question with the question of whether ignorance or knowledge would make for a better life for the physician if the physician were terminally ill. Nor must he confuse it with the question of whether the patient's life would be a *better life*—a life more valuable to others or to society—if it ended in ignorance rather than in truth. The question, rather, is whether it would be better *for the patient himself* to know or not to know his fate.

To judge that a certain ending of a life would be best for the person whose life it is, is to view that life as a unified process of development and to conclude that that ending is a fitting completion for that process. To view a human life as a unified process of development, however, is to view it selectively. Certain events or patterns of conduct are singled out as especially significant or valuable. To ascertain the best completion of a person's life for that person, then, is to make the most fundamental judgments about the value of that person's activities, aspirations, and experiences.

It might be replied that we do make such value judgments when we decide to end the physiologic life of a permanently comatose individual. In such cases we do make value judgments, but they are not judgments of this sort. On the contrary, we believe that since this individual's experience has ended, his life-process is already completed.

When the decision to withhold information of impending death is understood for what it is, it is difficult to see how anyone could presume to make it. My conjecture is that physicians are tempted to make these decisions in part because of a failure to reflect upon the disparity between two quite different kinds of judgments about what will harm or benefit the patient. Judgments of the first sort fall within the physician's competence as a highly trained medical expert. There is nothing in the physician's training which qualifies him to make judgments of the second sort—to evaluate another human being's life as a whole. Further, once the complexity of these judgments is appreciated and once their evaluative character is understood, it is implausible to hold that the physician is in a better position to make them than the patient or his family. The failure to ask what sorts of harm/benefit judgments may properly be made by the physician in his capacity as a physician is a fundamental feature of medical paternalism.

There is a more sophisticated version of the attempt to justify withholding of information in order to minimize harm to the patient or his family. This is the Contract Version of the Prevention of Harm Argument. The idea is that the physician-patient relationship is contractual and that the terms of this contract are such that the patient authorizes the physician to minimize harm to the patient (or his family) by whatever means he, the physician, deems necessary. Thus if the physician believes that the best way to minimize harm to the patient is to withhold information from him, he may do so without thereby wronging the patient. To wrong the patient the physician would either have to do something he was not authorized to do or fail to do something it was his duty to do and which was in his power to do. But in withholding information from the patient he is doing just what he is authorized to do. So he does the patient no wrong.

First of all, it should be noted that this version is vulnerable to the same objections just raised against the non-contractual Argument from the Prevention of Harm. The most serious of these is that in the cases of paternalism under discussion it is very doubtful that the physician will or even could possess the psychiatric and moral knowledge required for a well-founded judgment about what will be least harmful to the patient. In addition, the Contract Version is vulnerable to other objections. Consider the claim that the patient-physician relationship is a contract in which the patient authorizes the physician to prevent or minimize harm by whatever means the physician deems necessary, including the withholding of information. This claim could be interpreted in either of two ways: as a descriptive generalization about the way physicians and patients actually understand their relationship or as a normative claim about the way the physician-patient relationship should be viewed or may be viewed.

As a descriptive generalization it is certainly implausible—there are many people who do not believe they have authorized their physician to withhold the truth from them, and the legal doctrine of informed consent supports their view. Let us suppose for a moment that some people do view their relationship to their physician as including such an authorization and that there is nothing morally wrong with such a contract so long as both parties entered into it voluntarily and in full knowledge of the terms of the agreement.

Surely the fact that some people are willing to authorize physicians to withhold information from them would not justify the physician in acting toward other patients as if they had done so. The physician can only justify withholding information from a particular patient if this sort of contract was entered into freely and in full knowledge *by* *this* patient.

What, then, is the physician to do? Surely he cannot simply assume that all of his patients have authorized him to withhold the truth if he deems it necessary. Yet if in each case he inquires as to whether the patient wishes to make such an authorization, he will defeat the purpose of the authorization by undermining the patient's trust.

There is, however, a more serious difficulty. Even the more extreme advocates of medical paternalism must agree that there are some limits on the contractual relationship between physician and patient. Hence the obligations of each party are conditional upon the other party's observing the limits of the contract. The law, the medical profession, and the general public generally recognize that there are such limits. For example, the patient may refuse to undergo a certain treatment, he may seek a second opinion, or he may terminate the relationship altogether. Moreover, it is acknowledged that to decide to do any of these things the patient may—indeed perhaps must—rely on his own judgment. If he is conscientious he will make such decisions on consideration of whether the physician is doing a reasonable job of rendering the services for which he was hired.

There are general constraints on how those services may be rendered. If the treatment is unreasonably slow, if the physician's technique is patently sloppy, or if he employs legally questionable methods, the patient may rightly conclude that the physician has not lived up to the implicit terms of the agreement and terminate the relationship. There are also more special constraints on the contract stemming from the special nature of the problem which led the patient to seek the physician's services in the first place. If you go to a physician for treatment of a skin condition, but he ignores that problem and sets about trying to convince you to have cosmetic nose surgery, you may rightly terminate the relationship. These general and special constraints are limits on the agreement from the patient's point of view.

Now once it is admitted that there are any such terms—that the contract does have some limits and that the patient has the right to terminate the relationship if these limits are not observed by the physician—it must also be admitted that the patient must be in a position to discover *whether* those limits are being observed. But if the patient were to authorize the physician to withhold information, he might deprive himself of information which is relevant to determining whether the physician has observed the limits of the agreement.

I am not concerned to argue that authorizing a physician to withhold information is logically incompatible with the contract being conditional. My point, rather, is that to make such an authorization would show either that (a) one did not view the contract as being conditional or that (b) one did not take seriously the possibility that the conditions of the contract might be violated or that (c) one simply did not care whether the conditions were violated. Since it is unreasonable to expect a patient to make an unconditional contract or to ignore the possibility that conditions of the contract will be violated, and since one typically does care whether these conditions are observed, it is unreasonable to authorize the physician to withhold information when he sees fit. The Contract Version of the Argument from the Prevention of Harm, then, does not appear to be much of an improvement over its simpler predecessor.

There is one paternalist argument in favor of withholding of information which remains to be considered. This may be called the Argument from the Inability to Understand. The main premise is that the physician is justified in withholding information when the patient or his family is unable to understand the information. This argument is often used to justify paternalistic policies toward parents of defective infants in neonate intensive care units. The idea is that either their lack of intelligence or their excited emotional condition prevents parents from giving informed consent because they are incapable of being adequately informed. In such cases, it is said, "the doctrine of informed consent does not apply."[12]

This argument is also vulnerable to several objections. First, it too relies upon dubious and extremely broad psychological generalizations —in this case psychological generalizations about the cognitive powers of parents of defective neonates.

Second, and more importantly, it ignores the crucial question of the character of the institutional context in which parents find themselves. To the extent that paternalist attitudes shape medical institutions, this bleak estimate of the parental capacity for comprehension and rational decision tends to be a self-fulfilling prophecy. In an institution in which parents routinely sign operation permits without even having seen their newborn infants and without having the nature of the therapeutic options clearly explained to them, parents may indeed be incapable of understanding the little that they are told.

Third, it is a mistake to maintain that the legal duty to seek informed consent applies only where the physician can succeed in adequately informing parents. The doctor does not and cannot have a duty to make sure that all the information he conveys is understood by those to whom he conveys it. His duty is to make a reasonable effort to be understood.[13]

Fourth, it is important to ask exactly why it is so important not to tell parents information which they allegedly will not understand. If the reason is that a parental decision based on inadequate understanding will be a decision that is harmful to the *infant*, then the

12. Duff and Campbell, "Moral and Ethical Dilemmas," p. 893.
13. I would like to thank John Dolan for clarifying this point.

Argument from the Inability to Understand is not an argument for paternalism toward *parents*. So if this argument is to provide a justification for withholding information from parents for *their* benefit, then the claim must be that their failure to understand will somehow be harmful to *them*. But why should this be so? If the idea is that the parents will not only fail to understand but become distressed because they realize that they do not understand, then the Argument from the Inability to Understand turns out not to be a new argument at all. Instead, it is just a restatement of the Argument from the Prevention of Harm examined above—and is vulnerable to the same objections. I conclude that none of the three justifications examined provide adequate support for the paternalist practices under consideration. If adequate justification is to be found, the advocate of medical paternalism must marshal more powerful arguments.

V

So far I have examined several specific medical paternalist practices and criticized some general arguments offered in their behalf. Medical paternalism, however, goes much deeper than the specific practices themselves. For this reason I have spoken of "the medical paternalist model," emphasizing that what is at issue is a paradigm, a way of conceiving the physician-patient relationship. Indirect evidence for the pervasiveness of this model is to be found in the very words we use to describe physicians, patients, and their interactions. Simply by way of illustration, I will now examine one widely used distinction which expresses and helps perpetuate the paternalist model: the distinction between "ordinary" and "extraordinary" therapeutic measures.

Many physicians, theologians, ethicists, and judges have relied on this distinction since Pius XII employed it in an address on "The Prolongation of Life" in 1958. In reply to questions concerning conditions under which physicians may discontinue or refrain from initiating the use of artificial respiration devices, Pius first noted that physicians are duty-bound "to take the necessary treatment for the preservation of life and health." He then distinguished between "ordinary" and "extraordinary" means.

But normally one is held to use only ordinary means—according to circumstances of persons, places, times, and culture—means that do not involve any grave burden for oneself or another.[14]

Though he is not entirely explicit about this, Pius assumes that it is the right of the physician to determine what will count as "ordinary" or "extraordinary" means in any particular case.

In the context of the issue of when a highly trained specialist is to employ sophisticated life-support equipment, it is natural to assume that the distinction between "ordinary" and "extraordinary" means is a distinction between higher and lower degrees of technological sophistication. The Pope's unargued assumption that the medical specialist is to determine what counts as "ordinary" or "extraordinary" reinforces a technological interpretation of the distinction. After all, if the distinction is a technological one, then it is natural to assume that it is the physician who should determine its application since it is he who possesses the requisite technical expertise. In my discussions with physicians, nurses, and hospital administrators I have observed that they tend to treat the distinction as a technological one and then to argue that since it is a technological distinction the physician is the one who should determine in any particular case whether a procedure would involve "ordinary" or "extraordinary" means.[15]

Notice, however, that even though Pius introduced the distinction in the context of the proper use of sophisticated technical devices and even though he assumed that it was to be applied by those who possess the technical skills to use such equipment, it is quite clear that the distinction he explicitly introduced is not itself a technological distinction. Recall that he defines "ordinary" means as those which "do not involve any grave burden for oneself or another." "Extraordinary" means, then, would be those which do involve a grave burden for oneself or for another.

If what counts as "extraordinary" measures depended only upon

14. Pius XII, "The Prolongation of Life," in Reiser et al., *Ethics in Medicine*, (Cambridge, MA: MIT Press, 1977), pp. 501-504.

15. These discussions occurred in the course of my work as a member of committee which drafted ethical guidelines for Children's Hospital of Minneapolis.

what would constitute a "grave burden" to the patient himself, it might be easier to preserve the illusion that the decision is an exercise of medical expertise. But once the evaluation of burdens is extended to the patient's family it becomes obvious that the judgment that a certain therapy would be "extraordinary" is not a technological or even a clinical, but rather a *moral* decision. And it is a moral decision regardless of whether the evaluation is made from the perspective of the patient's own values and preferences or from that of the physician.

Even if one is to evaluate only the burdens for the patient himself, however, it is implausible to maintain that the application of the distinction is an exercise of technological or clinical judgment. For as soon as we ask what would result in "grave burdens" for the patient, we are immediately confronted with the task of making moral distinctions and moral evaluations concerning the quality of the patient's life and his interests as a person.

When pressed for an explanation of how physicians actually apply the distinction between "ordinary" and "extraordinary" therapeutic measures, the director of a neonate intensive care unit explained to me that what counts as "ordinary" or "extraordinary" differs in "different contexts." Surgical correction of a congenital gastrointestinal blockage in the case of an otherwise normal infant would be considered an "ordinary" measure. But the same operation on an infant with Downs' syndrome would be considered extraordinary.

I am not concerned here to criticize the moral decision to refrain from aggressive surgical treatment of infants with Down's syndrome. My purpose in citing this example is simply to point out that this decision *is* a moral decision and that the use of the distinction between "ordinary" and "extraordinary" measures does nothing to help one make the decision. The use of the distinction does accomplish something though: it obscures the fact that the decision *is* a moral decision. Even worse, it is likely to lead one to mistake a very controversial moral decision for a "value-free" technological or clinical decision. More importantly, to even suggest that a complex moral judgment is a clinical or technological judgment is to prejudice the issue of *who* has the right to decide whether life-sustaining measures are to be initiated or continued. Once controversial moral decisions are misperceived as clinical or technological decisions it becomes much easier for the medical paternalist to use the three arguments examined above to justify the withholding of information. For once it is conceded that his medical expertise gives the physician the right to make certain decisions, he can then argue that he may withhold information where this is necessary for the effective exercise of this right. By disguising complex moral judgments as medical judgments, then, the "ordinary/extraordinary" distinction reinforces medical paternalism.

VI

In this paper I have attempted to articulate and challenge some basic features of the medical paternalist model of the physician-patient relationship. I have also given an indication of the powerful influence this model exerts on medical practice and on ways of talking and thinking about medical treatment.

There are now signs that medical paternalism is beginning to be challenged from within the medical profession itself.[16] This, I believe, is all to the good. So far, however, challenges have been fragmentary and unsystematic. If they are to be theoretically and practically fruitful they must be grounded in a systematic understanding of what medical paternalism is and in a critical examination of justifications for medical paternalist practices. The present paper is an attempt to begin the task of such a systematic critique.

16. See, for example, A. Waldman, "Medical Ethics and the Hopelessly Ill Child," *The Journal of Pediatrics* 88, no. 5 (1976): 890-892.

I would like to thank Rolf Sartorius and the editors of *Philosophy & Public Affairs* for several helpful comments on an earlier draft of this paper.

A revised version of this article will appear in *Paternalism*, ed. Rolf E. Sartorious, forthcoming from the University of Minnesota Press.

DONALD VANDEVEER The Contractual Argument
for Withholding
Medical Information

Paternalistic grounds for justifying presumptively wrongful treatment
of competent adults are widely looked upon as suspect. Allen Buchanan, in an instructive and generally careful essay, has shown that
the presence of paternalistic attitudes and paternalistic treatment is
not uncommon in physicians' dealings with their patients.[1] In particular he contends that "the practice of withholding the truth from
the patient or his family, a particular form of medical paternalism, is
not adequately supported by the arguments advanced to justify it"
(p. 214). Buchanan distinguishes two types of arguments which may
be advanced against paternalism. The first sort would appeal to a
theory of moral rights and would seek (I presume, although Buchanan does not say so explicitly) to show that instances of medical
paternalism unjustifiably infringe one or more rights of the patient.
Assuming the absence of an adequate defense of a full-blown theory
of moral rights Buchanan prefers to advance an alternative critique.
He seeks to show that "paternalist justifications which are actually
employed by the practitioners of medical paternalism" are inadequate (p. 214). Contrary to Buchanan's claims I shall show that (1)
his attack on one attempt to justify the physician's withholding of information in a restricted range of cases is wrongheaded and that
there is in fact a strong presumption that it is permissible, and (2)
the physician's withholding information in these cases is not appropriately described as "medical paternalism."

1. Allen Buchanan, "Medical Paternalism" *Philosophy & Public Affairs* 7, no.
4 (Summer 1978): 370-390, and above, pp. 214-234. Page numbers in the text
refer to this article.

I

Buchanan observes that paternalism is usually characterized as "interference with a person's liberty of action, where the alleged justification of the interference is that it is for the good of the person whose liberty is thus restricted" (p. 215). Regarding the focus on liberty of *action* as too narrow, he prefers to include the withholding of information under similar conditions as also an instance of paternalistic interference. The characterization of paternalism is thus revised to include "interference with a person's freedom of action or freedom of information, or the deliberate dissemination of misinformation" (p. 215). I shall not object here to this extension of the more usual characterization.

After instructively documenting a tendency among physicians to attempt to justify withholding, or even falsifying, diagnostic information from their patients, Buchanan attempts to show the inadequacy of three arguments advanced to defend such practices. My focus will be solely on what he labels "the Contractual Version of Prevention of Harm Argument" (p. 221). It is worth quoting here his formulation of what I shall henceforth refer to as the Contractual Argument:

> The idea is that the physician-patient relationship is contractual and that the terms of this contract are such that the patient authorizes the physician to minimize harm to the patient (or his family) by whatever means he, the physician, deems necessary. Thus if the physician believes that the best way to minimize harm to the patient is to withhold information from him, he may do so without thereby wronging the patient. To wrong the patient the physician would either have to do something he was not authorized to do or fail to do something it was his duty to do and which was in his power to do. But in withholding information from the patient he is doing just what he is authorized to do. So he does the patient no wrong [p. 227].

Buchanan raises a series of objections against this argument. The first is one that may be brought against the claim that the physician may and ought to treat the patient in whatever way will be "least harmful" even in cases where there is no contractual agreement as described above. So a physician may legitimately withhold diagnostic information if he deems it the least harmful course of action. Buchanan objects that "it is very doubtful that the physician will or even could possess the psychiatric and moral knowledge required for a well-founded judgment about what will be least harmful for the patient" (p. 227). Elsewhere he emphasizes that a physician's judgments about certain matters are problematic—for example, when the judgment is made that a patient is likely to become fearful and develop a despondency which may progress into depressive illness (or culminate in suicide) if certain information is revealed to him (say he has terminal cancer). Such judgments, in Buchanan's view, involve *psychiatric generalizations* made typically on the basis of scanty evidence. He claims, further, that *even if* a physician is in a position to reliably predict, he may simply be assuming that suicide "is not a rational choice" for the patient (p. 223). Buchanan is correct, I believe, in judging that the physician who decides to withhold information on such grounds must make difficult empirical judgments and also difficult evaluative judgments about which alternative will be "least harmful" on balance for the patient. Several points, however, seriously weaken Buchanan's first objection to the Contractual Argument. Buchanan's reservations, if correct, serve only as a counsel of caution to the conscientious physician who wants to do what is least harmful to the patient. They do not show that it is impossible for a physician to arrive at a reasonable judgment that withholding information will be least harmful to the patient. Second, a physician may be in no more difficult position to make this judgment than the patient himself. Physicians are more likely, on average, than patients to have had training in psychiatric or psychological theory relevant to predicting the consequences of revealing disturbing information to patients. Further, they are more likely to have observed the effects of doing so in a wide variety of cases than laypersons. More significant, perhaps, is the point that as the Contract Argument is described, the patient has authorized the physician to minimize harm to the patient by *whatever means the physician deems necessary*. The contract is not and could not plausibly be one where the physician is authorized to act only on *correct* judgments. It must be an authorization for the physician to act only on the basis of what *he believes to be* a well-founded judgment. If the physician does so, he does not violate the terms of the contract *even if*, as it turns out, his judgment is not well-founded. That such judgments are difficult to make or that a physician may have failed to make one would not, thereby, show that he has done a wrong to his patient. An unwise judgment is not necessarily an unconscientious, negligent, or reckless one.

A second objection proposed by Buchanan is that not all patients understand their relationship with their physician to be one where they have authorized him (or her) to withhold information when deemed necessary to minimize harm (p. 228). So the physician, it is implied, cannot assume the existence of such a contract with a particular patient unless it is clear that *this* patient has contracted freely and with full knowledge that he has done so. These points are surely correct. It should be clear, however, that neither supposition undermines the Contractual Argument for it purports to justify withholding information *only* when there *is* a contractual authorization to do so. Again, we can only advise caution for physicians who may be tempted to assume authorization when there is inadequate reason to make such an assumption. Buchanan's claims may also be taken to urge patients to make explicit agreements with physicians so that there are no false or unfounded assumptions about the reciprocal rights and duties of the contracting parties. Since such matters are often not well defined, the point is well taken. Once more, it does not strike a blow against the Contractual Argument.

Buchanan presses his point further by claiming that if the physician inquires in each case whether the patient wishes to authorize the withholding of certain information "he will defeat the purpose of the authorization by undermining the patient's trust" (p. 231). If correct this claim shows, not that the Contractual Argument is unsound, but that such contracting is not likely to occur or that there is a reason to avoid forming such contracts. Hence, claims that such a contract was agreed upon ought to be viewed skeptically. The claim that such inquiries do or would undermine the patient's trust is itself, I think, a dubious empirical generalization although I cannot disprove it. A patient asked by his physician if he wishes to have possibly disturbing diagnostic information withheld from him when the physician may judge its revelation harmful to him would be inclined to judge that his physician is conscientious and principled, that he is a person unwilling to treat a patient in a presumptively wrong manner in the absence of his express consent to such a policy. Such an inquiry would tend to confirm a patient's hope that his physician respects the patient's right to decide how he shall be treated and will not treat him in a suspect way just because the physician judges it to be "for the patient's own good." That is, the inquiry would support the claim that the physician was *not* a member of the fraternity of paternalists.

Buchanan claims, however, that there is yet "a more serious difficulty" (p. 228). He states that even extreme advocates of medical paternalism must agree that there must be some limits on the contractual relationship between patient and physician. In particular, the patient needs to be able to determine whether the physician is observing the limitations imposed by the contractual relationship. If the patient authorizes the physician to withhold information he may deprive himself of the information necessary to determine *whether or not* those limits are being observed. In Buchanan's view such an authorization would show that "(a) one did not view the contract as being conditional or that (b) one did not take seriously the possibility that the conditions of the contract might be violated or that (c) one simply did not care whether the conditions were violated" (p. 229). Thus, it is concluded that it is unreasonable to authorize the physician to withhold information when he sees fit. There are difficulties with this line of thought. Surely, it cannot be maintained that the patient should do nothing which would make it impossible or difficult to determine whether contractual limits are being observed. If so, the patient would never submit to anesthesia which would, after all, impair his ability to oversee a surgeon's procedure. More importantly it is possible that a patient might authorize the withholding of information and yet the conditions mentioned in (a), (b), and (c) are not true of the patient. For example, I might want certain information revealed to me and other information not revealed. Recognizing the benefits frequently associated with the "placebo effect" I may reasonably prefer not to be told when a placebo has been prescribed as part of my treatment. Also, I may recognize my penchant for undue anxi-

ety and worry over the fact that certain of my symptoms are suggestive but not conclusive evidence of the presence of some dreaded
disease. Hence, I may choose to remain ignorant of such matters until
the physician is certain of its presence. Further, if my affairs are in
order, I may even prefer to live out my last days falsely hopeful of re-
covery even when the physician is certain that I have terminal cancer.
These preferences for ignorance with regard to a certain range of
information may be made clear to the physician in a contract. With
regard to certain matters I may authorize the physician to use his best
judgment about whether it will be least harmful to disclose or to withhold information. Ignorance is not always bliss, but an individual
may prefer ignorance under certain conditions. The nature of the
contract made would obviously depend on one's preferences and one's
degree of trust and confidence in the judgment in one's physician.

Thus, whether or not the physician wrongfully withholds information will depend on the nature of the contract. It may authorize and
require disclosure of certain information *and also* authorize and require the withholding of other information. An interesting result
shows up here. If I contract *not* to be informed of terminal cancer
should I have it and the physician later decides that my *not* being informed of this fact is more harmful to me on balance than my being
informed and he thus informs me, his *disclosure* would be *paternalistic interference* with my chosen course, with my freedom to choose
what information I shall receive. Hence, it is misleading to focus
solely on the cases of withholding information or giving misinformation proceeding from paternalistic motives as actions requiring justification. Disclosing information may also be a paternalistic act and,
possibly, an unjustifiable form of paternalism.

Buchanan maintains that "it is unreasonable to authorize the physician to withhold information when he sees fit" (p. 229). If he means
"whenever, without qualification," I certainly agree. I have tried to
show how it may be reasonable to authorize withholding information
on certain matters. Hence, withholding information need not be
paternalistic interference, and, indeed, disclosure may be. That depends on the nature of the contract, whether its authorizations are
reasonable or not.

II

In view of the preceding remarks my second basic point can be defended more briefly. It is that in a certain range of cases where the physician withholds information from the patient, we do not have a case of medical paternalism. Hence, a justification for doing so is not a justification of medical paternalism.

As noted earlier, since Buchanan regards the (partial) characterization of paternalism as interference with "freedom of action" as too narrow, he expands the characterization to include "freedom of information, or the deliberate dissemination of misinformation" (p. 216). For reasons mentioned "freedom of information" may be understood to mean "freedom to be provided with information" or "freedom to not be subjected to information." Whether the disclosure of information or its being withheld is an *interference* depends on whether what the physician does violates the terms of the contract which, if well-made, will express the patient's preference for ignorance or disclosure, or some combination thereof. Hence, what the patient prefers and consents to is a crucial determinant in deciding whether a physician *interferes* with the patient, and, therefore, whether the physician *paternalistically interferes* with the patient. If a patient contracts to authorize his physician to withhold information under certain conditions, then the physician's doing so *under those conditions* is not a case of interference and, hence, not paternalistic interference.[2] It is rather a case of compliance with the terms of the contract and not appropriately adduced as an instance of "medical paternalism." The withholding of information in such a case may even be an act the physician reluctantly agrees to but, in order to respect his *patient's* judgment about what is "for his (the patient's) own good," he complies with such a wish. So the withholding of information need not be paternalistic at all and, if it is justified, may be justified because it is the honoring of a contractual agreement, a respecting of the patient's autonomy rather than an overriding or disregarding of it.

If my arguments succeed, they are of course compatible with the

2. I elaborate on the relation of prior consent to paternalistic interference in a forthcoming essay in the *Canadian Journal of Philosophy*, "Paternalism and Subsequent Consent."

overly neglected fact that medical paternalism is not uncommon and that purported justifications of it bear critical attention. If such paternalism is suspect, as I believe, it is important to identify ways of minimizing or avoiding it. In fact the making of explicit contracts with adequate checks on compliance by both parties seems just such a way of doing so. Whether any particular physician-patient relationship involves a contract of this more or less ideal sort is an empirical question about which I have avoided generalizing. A purported justification of a particular withholding of information may fail in its appeal to contractual authorization to do so simply because there has been no such contractual authorization. The remedy for practices lacking such authorization may be an increased turn toward the making of such contracts. The Contractual Argument, then, proffers not a justification of paternalistic interference, but rather a non-paternalistic justification of treating patients in ways that, abstractly considered, would be judged presumptively wrong. As such it is not vulnerable to the sorts of objections which may be brought against purported justifications of genuinely paternalistic treatment of patients.

PART IV
Euthanasia

JOEL FEINBERG

Voluntary Euthanasia and the Inalienable Right to Life

It is surprising that in this bicentennial period we have not yet heard an argument that seems to bolster the case of opponents of voluntary euthanasia. The argument derives from an interpretation of Thomas Jefferson's famous words that all men "are endowed by their Creator with certain unalienable Rights, that among these are Life . . . ," and from similar passages in the writings of other founding fathers. To kill another person even with his consent or at his considered request, it might well be claimed, is to infringe his "Right to Life," a right the founders clearly held to be incapable of being waived or surrendered. Willfully to take one's own life or to permit another to take one's life, the argument continues, is in the relevant sense to *alienate* one's right to go on living; hence, suicide and voluntary euthanasia can both be viewed as efforts to alienate the inalienable, to give away what cannot properly be given away.

There is at least a superficial plausibility in this effort to invoke the authority of Jefferson as a basis for refusing legal sanction or denying moral legitimacy to such practices as suicide, aiding another's suicide, and voluntary euthanasia. The argument seems to present a dilemma for those of us who would defend a "right to die": either we must abandon our defense of what seem to us to be morally justifiable practices, or else we must reject the exalted eighteenth-century doctrine of inalienable rights, at least as it applies to the right to life. The former alternative seems inhumane and paternalistic, the latter seems virtually un-American. I have my doubts about the theory of inalienable rights in any case—doubts that will emerge in the following discussion —but my primary intention in this essay is to find a way between two alternatives by reconciling a right to die with the inalienability of the right to live, properly interpreted.

I. THE RIGHT TO LIFE

Just what kind of right is "the right to life"? Numerous distinctions can be made, of course, among the many types and categories of rights. While it is impossible here to work our way completely through the conceptual maze, it will be useful to clarify the right to life by placing it in relation to some of the more important of these distinctions. This will be in part a matter of stipulation, for the right to life is interpreted in different ways by different writers, and where there is disagreement or confusion, I can only try to make persuasive suggestions that one or another interpretation is more standard, useful, or important.

I propose, first of all, to interpret "the right to life" in a relatively narrow way, so that it refers to "the right not to be killed" and "the right to be rescued from impending death," but not to the broader conception, favored by many manifesto writers, of a "right to live decently." To be sure, as Hugo Bedau put it, ". . . the life to which we now think men are entitled as of right is not [merely] a right at the barest level sufficient to stave off an untimely death; rather it is a life sufficient for self-respect, relief from needless drudgery, and opportunity for the release of productive energy."[1] However, we can refer separately to the components of a right to live decently: a right to decent working conditions, a right to food, to clothing, to housing, to education, and so on. Another component right in this comprehensive package of rights is the right not to be killed or allowed to die. *This* is the right that is characteristically at issue in debates over euthanasia and suicide, not the various welfare rights enumerated in twentieth-

1. Hugo Bedau, "The Right to Life," *The Monist* 52 (1968): 567.

century manifestoes. It would ill serve clarity, therefore, to use the generic label when we are concerned only with the specific subspecies.

The right to life, in the second place, is generally thought, at least in our time, to be a *claim-right* as opposed to a right in the sense of mere liberty, privilege, or absence of duty to refrain. A claim-right is a more complex notion, and presumably a more valuable benefit, than a liberty. To say that John Doe is at liberty to do or have X is to say simply that he has no duty to refrain from or relinquish X. But that is not yet to say anything about anyone else's duties to Doe in respect to X. Doe may have a right (in the sense of liberty) to X even though everyone else is also at liberty to interfere with his efforts to do or possess X. If Doe's right to X, however, is a claim-right, then Doe is at liberty to do or have X, and his liberty is the ground of other people's duties either to grant him X or not to interfere with his doing or possessing X. A claim-right then is a liberty correlated with another person's duty (or *all* other persons' duties) not to interfere. If Doe has a claim-right to life, then those against whom he has the claim (presumably all the rest of us) have duties not to kill him or let him die when we can save him with no danger to ourselves. If, on the other hand, Doe's right to life were a mere liberty, it would amount to no more than the absence of a duty to kill or to fail to save himself, an absence that is perfectly consistent with the liberties and even the duties of others to kill him.

Even a "liberty-right" to life, while not as comfortable a protection as a claim-right, has some importance. Indeed, Thomas Hobbes interpreted the right to defend one's life as a "natural liberty," and made it the foundation of his political philosophy. In a state of nature there are no duties, hence everyone has complete liberty. The natural liberty to defend one's own life (that is, the absence of a duty to cooperate in one's own extinction) is so very important to everyone's natural interest and basic motivation, Hobbes thought, that no one in his right mind would ever agree to bargain it away in the negotiations that lead to the creation of civil society with its complex of new duties and claim-rights. Indeed, the strengthening of personal security is the essence of civil society, the "name of its game." Not even a prisoner convicted of a capital crime acquires a duty to cooperate with his executioner, though of course the latter will have the liberty, the duty, and the power to execute him in the name of the state.[2] The Hobbesian "natural liberty" guarantees that one can never have the duty to die; the "right to life" in the sense here being explained, in contrast, guarantees that (under normal conditions at least) others cannot be at liberty to kill you.

To have a right, then, is to have a claim against others, and claims can be further distinguished in terms of their *addressees*. The right to life, as we shall understand it here, is a *double-barreled* claim, addressed to two distinct sets of claimees. On the one hand, it is a right *in rem* holding against the "world at large," or all other private individuals or groups that might ever be in a position to kill or fail to save the claimant. On the other hand, it is (or ought to be) a claim that its possessor can make against the state for its legal enforcement. The former set of claims, being based on reasons derived from moral principles, are binding on the consciences of other persons and are the grounds of their duties to rescue or to forbear killing the claimant. As such, these claims can exist prior to or independently of their recognition by the state. Hence, they are, in the appropriate sense, *moral rights*. When they are recognized by the state they acquire support from reasons of an additional kind derived from legal rules and thus become legal claim-rights against one's fellow citizens, as well as moral rights. Enforcement-claims—which can have both a moral and a legal backing—obligate the state to require performance of the moral obligations that others have to me and to protect me by threat of punishment from wrongful interference. Valid laws often impose genuine obligations on the state (to refund excess tax payments, to provide trial by jury, to punish crimes, for example) and hence confer correlative rights of a legal kind on citizens as against the state. My (moral) right to life, however, would constitute a morally binding claim to enforcement against the state even in the fancifully hypothetical circumstance in which there were no laws against homicide. I

2. Stephen Becker's highly philosophical novel, *A Covenant With Death* (New York, 1965), tells of a relevant dilemma. A judge must decide the fate of a prisoner, wrongly convicted of murder, who kills the hangman lawfully attempting his execution. The judge decides to follow Hobbes and declares the prisoner not guilty of any crime.

would in that case have a powerful claim against the legislature to *make* laws against homicide so that the moral right to life would be converted into a legal right as well. In actual, prevailing circumstances, I have a moral (but not legal) claim-right against the Congress not to be victimized by the passage into law of invidious, though constitutional, legislation.

The right to life, as I shall understand it here, also belongs to that subclass of moral rights that are said, in virtue of their fundamentally important, indeed essential, connection with human well-being, to belong equally and unconditionally to all human beings, simply in virtue of their being human. It is, therefore, what the United Nations called a *human right*.[3] There is a controversy among philosophers whether all, or even any, human rights are *absolute rights*. That dispute is far too complicated to resolve here, but it will be useful to show in a sketchy way its bearing on the concept of a right to life. An absolute right (if there is such a thing) is a right that would remain in one's possession, fully effective as a ground for other people's duties to one, in all possible circumstances. If my right to X is absolute, then there are no circumstances in which it is "subject to legitimate limitation" or in which the correlated duties of others to me in respect to X are suspended. If the right is absolute, then I possess it, and others are bound to me in the appropriate ways in all circumstances *without exception*. This unqualified and exceptionless character of an absolute right implies (among other things) that it can never be in unresolved conflict with the absolute rights of other persons, whether those rights are of the same type (for example, rights to life) or of another type (say, rights to liberty or to property). If my right to life is absolute in this sense, and if my life can be saved only at the cost of taking your property, then your right to property cannot also be an absolute right, for it will be limited or suspended in this case of unavoidable conflict. In short, if conflicts occur between one person's absolute right and another person's right of another kind, the absolute right must always triumph. But it also follows that unavoidable conflict between one person's absolute right and another person's absolute right of the same type (for example, the right to life of two different persons) is

3. UNESCO, *Human Rights, a Symposium* (London and New York: Allan Wingate, 1949).

logically impossible in just the manner of a hypothetical conflict between an irresistible force and an immovable object. It simply cannot
happen.

Since conflicts between rights do occur, it is implausible to maintain
that *all* rights are absolute in the present sense. A more difficult question, indeed, is whether *any* rights at all can so qualify. In any event,
it seems very doubtful that the right to life, as it is normally understood, can be absolute. A great many people who profess a belief in
the right to life also support the killing of enemy combatants in war,
capital punishment of convicted murderers, and killing of assailants
and even "innocent aggressors" in self-defense. These people find no
conflict in maintaining that everyone has a right not to be killed ("the
right to life") while holding also that there are circumstances which
limit the application of that right and require its suspension. The
"right to life" that they believe in, therefore, cannot be absolute.

Nevertheless, it is hard to shed the intuitive conviction that there
is somehow *something* that is "absolute" in the natural or human right
to life (and the rights to liberty and property too, for that matter).
There are at least three strategies that have governed the efforts of
philosophers to isolate, specify, and strengthen that lingering intuition. Any one of the strategies would, if successful, be sufficient, but
in theory they might also be used in various combinations. The first
of these is the *method of presumptiveness*. One might conclude, with
William Frankena, that certain human rights, including the right to
life, are only prima facie rights.[4] That is, in every possible circumstance a person's right to life will be an actual right, commanding forbearance or performance from others, *except* where it is in unavoidable conflict with someone else's right to life (or to something else)
which happens to be more stringent in the circumstances. In that
unhappy situation the other party's actual right prevails and the
presumption that one has one's normal right to life in *that situation*,
as one does in most others, is overridden. But the presumptive right to
life, as a presumption, always holds. It is the prima facie right that
is absolute, not the actual right which may not be present in a rare
instance of conflict. To declare that all persons have absolute prima

4. W. K. Frankena, "Natural and Inalienable Rights," *Philosophical Review*
64 (1955).

facie rights to life and other goods is "to say that interfering with
[their] enjoyment of them always requires a moral justification."[5]
There is *always* a presumption of the existence of the actual right,
even though that presumption is not necessarily decisive in every possible situation. At least something, therefore, is constant and invariant
in all circumstances.

This position may be expressed more clearly by employing the distinction between having a right and having a claim. To have a claim
is to have reasons of some weight that put one in a position to make
claim to something.[6] These reasons support the claim and lend it
credence and cogency, even if, in the end, they should fail to *establish*
the claim and compel its recognition. Unlike rights, claims can differ
in degree: some are stronger than others. One very good kind of reason for denying that John Doe's admitted claim to X amounts to a
right to X in the present circumstances is that Richard Roe also has a
claim to X, and it is impossible for both Doe and Roe to do or have X.
In that case, Roe (at most) has the right to X; nevertheless, it remains
true that even in the circumstances that obtained, Doe did have a
strong, but not decisive, *claim.* Using this terminology, a philosopher
could affirm that *all persons always* have a powerful claim not to be
killed even in those tragic circumstances where it is outweighed by a
more powerful claim on the other side. If a judge or moral critic con-
cedes the existence of the powerful claim while denying that it
amounts to an actual right in the present circumstances, he thereby
assumes the burden of showing how it is outweighed and overridden
in the circumstances that prevail. Again *something* remains "absolute"
and constant, namely the existence of the claim.

The second strategy for preserving an absolute element can be
called, following Judith Thomson, the *method of full factual specification.*[7] A philosopher friendly to the idea of absolute human rights
might argue that all simple and brief statements of (say) the right to
life are of necessity mere abbreviations for an elaborately complex

5. Ibid., p. 228.
6. I have discussed this in Joel Feinberg, *Social Philosophy* (Englewood
Cliffs, N.J., 1973), p. 68.
7. Judith J. Thomson, "Self-defense and Rights," *The Lindley Lecture*, University of Kansas, 1976.

statement defining a right that *is* absolute. The fuller statement would begin, presumably, by stating that all "human beings" (a phrase itself in need of detailed definition) have a right not to be killed. It would then proceed to explain what is to be understood by "killing" and which circumstances—described in a general, but not *too* general, way—constitute exceptions (this could lead to a discussion of war, capital punishment, and self-defense, among other topics). The statement would include a discussion of what priority rules are to be used for determining who has the right and who does not in situations of unavoidable conflict; again, these rules would be described in a general, but not too general, way. A similarly detailed statement would follow, describing the full extent, within carefully circumscribed limits, of the right to be rescued. Clearly such an enterprise would yield a book-length statement at the very least. Philosophers who prefer the method of presumptiveness are pessimistic about the plausibility of doing this, even in principle, and defenders of the method of full factual specification would have to admit that it has not yet been done in fact.

A more difficult problem comes from the inevitable loss of any semblance of Jefferson's self-evident truths in such a statement. Most of us would affirm without hesitation our belief in a human right to life, but any fully specified statement of that right, including the *correct* one (assuming that there is in principle *one* correct one), would divide us into a hundred quarreling sects disputing such questions as abortion, capital punishment, and the like. It is doubtful that *any* fully specified declaration of a right to life could ever win the unanimous assent of all those who believe that the existence of such a right is obvious. What is self-evident, according to this second view of the matter, can only be a bare "lowest common denominator" of a large number of contending moral systems, perhaps no more than what I have called, with deliberate vagueness, "an ideal directive to legislative aspiration commanding us to do our best for the cause of human life as we judge the various claims that may be before us in our roles as legislators, judges, and moral agents."[8] Or perhaps the common ground includes more precise and significant areas. Com-

8. Feinberg, *Social Philosophy*, p. 71.

mon to the moral systems of all who profess belief in a human right to life, after all, are such judgments as: it is always wrong to shoot a normal adult human being in the back of the head for the purpose of taking his money to buy luxuries for one's own enjoyment. When we include some of the circumstances in the description of the act, we can say that the right not to be the victim of such an action holds "in all possible circumstances." Beyond such examples, the method of full factual specification permits us to say that other human rights, fully specified, are absolute, but only at the cost of admitting that we do not really know, and cannot agree, which rights exactly these are.

The third strategy, which I shall call the method of *justified infringement*, can coexist with either of the other two. No matter how we separate out actual rights from prima facie or presumptive rights, rights from claims, abbreviated statements of rights that are unqualified and thus not absolute from fully expanded statements of rights that are exceptionless, we must face the possibility that some quite actual rights that are possessed by their owners in all situations can nevertheless be rightly infringed in certain unusual circumstances. As Bedau puts it, "A person's possessing a right is not always dispositive of the issue of how he ought to be treated."[9] If it can make sense to speak of the justified invasion of a genuine actual right, a "justified injustice" as it were, then it will be possible to speak of the proper infringement of an absolute right (that is, a right which is held by its possessor in all circumstances). In that case, the doctrine of absolute rights can be preserved even in the face of convincing examples of justified treatment contrary to what the right, considered alone, would require. Absolute rights, of course, are claim-rights and therefore logically correlated with the *duties* of other people to perform or forbear as the right, considered alone, requires. Thus a logical consequence of the view that sometimes one may justifiably infringe another's right is the proposition that on occasion one may justifiably fail to discharge one's duty.

At this point, it will be useful to borrow Judith Thomson's distinction between infringing and violating a person's right: ". . . we *violate* his right if and only if we do not merely infringe it, but more, are

9. Bedau, "The Right to Life," p. 569.

acting wrongly, unjustly, in doing so. Now the view that rights are 'absolute' in the sense I have in mind is the view that every infringing of a right is a violating of a right."[10] We can readily provide examples of rights that are *not* absolute in Thomson's sense. Perhaps the most plausible of these are property rights. Suppose that you are on a back-packing trip in the high mountain country when an unanticipated blizzard strikes the area with such ferocity that your life is imperiled. Fortunately, you stumble onto an unoccupied cabin, locked and boarded up for the winter, clearly somebody else's private property. You smash in a window, enter, and huddle in a corner for three days until the storm abates. During this period you help yourself to your unknown benefactor's food supply and burn his wooden furniture in the fireplace to keep warm. Surely you are justified in doing all these things, and yet you have infringed the clear rights of another person.

It will be argued, on the other side, that you have not infringed any-one's actual rights that were fully operative in the circumstances but only prima facie rights, the overturned presumption of rights, or inconclusive claims. It will be said, perhaps, that the undeniable right of the homeowner, when fully specified, excludes emergency circum-stances such as the ones that obtained, and thus he can have no grievance or counterclaim against you. It is, of course, possible to *say* these things, but only at the cost of rejecting the way most of us actu-ally understand the rights in question. We would not think it inappro-priate to express our gratitude to the homeowner, after the fact, and our regrets for the damage we have inflicted on his property. More importantly, almost everyone would agree that you owe *compensation* to the homeowner for the depletion of his larder, the breaking of his window, and the destruction of his furniture. One owes compensation here for the same reason one must repay a debt or return what one has borrowed. If the other had no right that was infringed in the first place, one could hardly have a duty to compensate him. Perhaps he would be an appropriate object of your sympathy or patronage or charity, but those are quite different from compensation. This is a case, then, of the infringement but not the violation of a property right.

10. Thomson, "Self-defense and Rights."

Not every case of justified killing infringes the victim's right to life. We may still have to resort to the presumptiveness strategy or the full specification strategy to explain why we do not infringe the victim's right to life in war killing, capital punishment, or self-defense. The other's right to life may not extend as far as these cases of justified killing and hence may not be involved at all. Surely, we acknowledge no duty of compensation to the heirs of an aggressor whom we killed in self-defense. On the other hand, there are some rare cases, as Thomson points out, of justified killing of innocents whose rights to life *are* thereby infringed—"If you are an innocent threat to my life (you threaten it through no fault of your own), and I can save my life only by killing you, and therefore do kill you, I think I do owe compensation, for I take your life to save mine."[11] One of Thomson's examples of an innocent threat is an "innocent shield," a child tied to the front of a tank driven by a malevolent aggressor whose intent is clearly to destroy me. There is no place for me to hide, but I happen to have an antitank gun, so to save my own life I blow up the tank, killing both the wicked aggressor and the innocent child. Self-defense presumably justifies me, and I have no duty afterwards to compensate the aggressor, but the child's right has been infringed, and I would have a strong obligation to set things straight somehow with her parents. In her case, I have infringed a right to life without violating it, so her right to life was not "absolute" in Thomson's sense, but the example does not show that her right was not absolute in our original sense, for the right continued to exist even in the circumstance where it was justifiably infringed. The "absolute" element in the *aggressor's* general right to life, however, if there is such a thing at all, must be demonstrated by one of the first two methods.

We may now tentatively conclude that by "the right to life" we can mean a right not to be killed or allowed to die which can be claimed against all other private individuals and groups for their forbearance and performance, and against the state for its enforcement. As a claim-right it signifies not merely the absence of a duty to cooperate in one's own death, but also the correlative duties of others toward one. It is a moral right in the sense that it is a claim rendered valid by

11. Ibid.

reasons derived from moral principle, and therefore can exist prior to and independently of legal recognition. It is presumably a human right since it is thought to be possessed equally by all human beings simply in virtue of their being human. Put simply and unqualifiedly as the right not to be killed or allowed to die, it is generally thought *not* to be an absolute right, since there are circumstances in which some human beings—soldiers, convicted murderers, homicidal aggressors—seem to be without it. Many philosophers, however, have tried by one method or another to isolate something that subsists through all the circumstances in which a human being with a right to life might find himself. Some locate the invariant element in a standing presumption of a right (a "prima facie right") or a constant but rebuttable claim to life. Others interpret the right to life in the bare minimal formulation given here as a mere abbreviation for a complex statement full of conditions and exceptions that does define an absolute right. Still others point out that in difficult circumstances some very basic rights can be infringed without being violated, and while this shows that they are not "absolute" in one sense (Thomson's), it is a way of showing the persistence of the right in some situations that might otherwise be thought to be inconsistent with its absoluteness in our present sense of context-invariance.

II. Discretionary and Mandatory Rights

Up to this point the defining characteristics I have attributed to the right to life are either commonplace and uncontroversial or else technical and controverted only by abstract theorists. Now we come to a question about the right to life that is both controversial and directly relevant to our ulterior purposes. We must now ask how the distinction between "discretionary" and "mandatory" rights applies to the right to life. This is a familiar distinction which has borne a number of other names. Martin Golding has formulated it as well as any, using the terms "option-right" and "welfare-right."[12] A discretionary right, which

12. I have no quarrel with the label "option-right" and shall use it as an alternative way of referring to discretionary rights, but I find "welfare-rights" a misleading and even question-begging term insofar as it suggests that all of the rights we naturally associate with "welfare"—such as the right to a job, to medical care, to education—are necessarily what I call "mandatory rights."

Golding calls an option-right, is "an area of autonomy within which the right-holder alone is free to decide."[13] I have a discretionary right in respect to X when I have an *open option* to X or not to X correlated with the duties of others not to interfere with my choice. It is important to note that if I have a discretionary right to do X, it follows logically that I have a right also not to do X, if I should so choose. It cannot be the case that my right leaves me free to X but not free not to X. Any discretionary right to something is a right to take it or leave it, as one chooses. A mandatory right, in contrast, confers no discretion whatever on its possessor: only one way of exercising it is permitted. It leaves one path open to him but no genuine "option" between paths. It imposes a correlative duty on others to provide that path and leave it unobstructed, but it imposes no duty upon others of noninterference with deviance from the single permitted track. If I have a mandatory right to do X then it follows logically that I have—not a right not to do X—but rather a *duty* to do X. In the case of mandatory rights, duty and right are entirely coincident.

Golding cites the right to education as his chief example of a mandatory right. All children in a certain age group have a right to attend a school and receive instruction from teachers in it. At the same time, those children, since school attendance is required, have a *duty* to attend school. The right and the duty coincide; there is no free play for "discretion"; therefore, the right is mandatory.

Very likely there is no gainsaying Golding on his account of the right to education, but to those who find the very idea of a mandatory right intolerably paradoxical there is one possible way out. That is to interpret the right as a claim that each citizen has to live in an educated society. On this construction, each person has a right that all the *other* persons be educated, and in virtue of the right that the others have that *he* be educated, he has himself a duty to attend school. It is because of other people's rights that he has a duty to go to school, not because of his own. If he has no discretion in the matter, that is because the discretion theoretically lies with the others to release him or hold him to his duty. This is a perfectly coherent account of something to which "the right to education" might refer and, so interpreted,

13. Martin P. Golding, "Towards a Theory of Human Rights," *The Monist* 52 (1968): 546.

the right to education is not quite the same thing as a mandatory right. The only trouble with it is that it is not a very accurate account of what most of us mean in ordinary political discourse when we speak of "the right to education." We ordinarily have in mind, when we use that phrase, a claim that each child can make to his *own* education, not merely, or not only, a claim that he can make to be a member of an educated community.

Still, it is easy to understand why people should be uneasy with the very idea of a mandatory right. The theory behind the idea seems to be that there are certain undeniable benefits, such as education, health, welfare, to which we are all entitled, and that these benefits are so important that it cannot be in anybody's interest ever to forgo them. Opportunity to enjoy these benefits must be provided by others and not interfered with by others; because the benefits are undeniably advantageous whatever the beneficiary may think about the matter, the latter must not be free to forgo them. The concept of a mandatory right, in short, would seem to be a paternalistic notion, reasonably enough applied to children, but offensively demeaning when imposed on presumably autonomous adults. Perhaps that is why Golding's most plausible example of such a right, the right to education, is one thought by most of us to apply (at least in its mandatory aspect) to children only. Another perennial philosophical candidate for such a status is the "right to punishment" conferred by righteous moralizers on qualified wrongdoers in the same condescending spirit as that with which the nurse gives the reluctant child his evil-tasting medicine. ("*We* know that, unpleasant as it may seem, this treatment is bound to do you more good than harm in the long run. In fact, it is what you *need* if you are to get better, and you must take it if only for your own sake.") The contrast with option-rights, which we are free to exercise as we please, is striking in this respect. The primary benefit conferred by a discretionary right is a certain amount of guaranteed freedom; mandatory rights are guaranteed opportunities to secure goods of other kinds (education, moral regeneration, health) that are paid for by sacrifices of freedom.

The idea of a mandatory right, moreover, brings to mind some frightful sophistries. We recall the odious arguments used throughout history both by revolutionaries and reactionaries that there can be freedom to do good but not to do evil, to speak truth but not falsehood, to worship true but not false gods. "Freedom" to do evil, to speak falsehood, to commit religious error, is not freedom at all, it is said, but mere license. From this, it is but a short step to the view expressed in what Isaiah Berlin calls a typical statement made by a Jacobin club during the Terror: "No man is free in doing evil. To prevent him is to set him free."[14] Then if we guarantee a Jacobin "freedom" by imposing duties of noninterference on others enforced by the state, we have converted it into a "mandatory right."

Still, in all fairness, there is no necessity that any given mandatory right be enmeshed in such specious rhetoric. A mandatory right, after all, is a kind of duty looked at in a certain positive way, and there need be nothing sinister in the assignment of duties to people. Every duty trivially entails a liberty to do what duty requires. (A liberty to do X being defined as the *absence of a duty not* to do X.) When it is vitally important and essentially advantageous not only to the community in general but to the moral agent himself that his duty be discharged, we are likely to guarantee him, by the imposition of duties of noninterference on others, the opportunity to do his duty. Then the liberty trivially entailed by duty takes on the appearance of a claim-right against others. If the personal and social interest in the successful performance of the duty is great enough, opportunity to perform is guaranteed, opportunity to fail to perform is totally withdrawn, and, at this point, enforcible duty, treasured opportunity, and claim-right all coalesce into mandatory right. (All that is missing to the possessor is freedom.) Many duties are onerous burdens that, no matter how heavy, must be carried and many yield benefits to the bearer that he will surely wish to reap. Whether we describe these hybrids as duties or rights will depend on whether we wish to emphasize their character as hardships or benefits; on whether our aim is to threaten and entreat, or persuade and induce. Hegelian moralists describe the convicted criminal's duty to submit to punishment as a "right to be punished" when they wish to emphasize that punishment can provide

14. Sir Isaiah Berlin, *Four Essays on Liberty* (New York, 1969), p. 148 n.

the criminal with a unique opportunity for moral regeneration, a state of being that would be truly beneficial to him, whether he knows it now or not.

However, we do not have to think of duties that are hidden or of benefits that are unsuspected to appreciate the present point. Many of the most ordinary and often irksome political duties are easily conceived, without paradox, as genuine benefits; they are ardently pursued and demanded as rights by those who are not permitted to qualify for them. In Tolstoy's *Anna Karenina*, a group of country gentry discussing women's liberation come to an appreciation of the point quite naturally:

> Alexey Alexandrovitch expressed the idea that the education of women is apt to be confounded with the emancipation of women, and it is only so that it can be considered dangerous.
>
> "I consider, on the contrary, that the two questions are inseparably connected together," said Pestov; "it is a vicious circle. Woman is deprived of rights from lack of education, and the lack of education results from the absence of rights. We must not forget that the subjection of women is so complete, and dates from such ages back that we are often unwilling to recognize the gulf that separates them from us," said he.
>
> "You said rights," said Sergey Ivanovitch, waiting till Pestov had finished, "meaning the right of sitting on juries, of voting, of presiding at official meetings, the right of entering the civil service, of sitting in parliament . . ."
>
> "Undoubtedly."
>
> "But if women, as a rare exception, can occupy such positions, it seems to me you are wrong in using the expression 'rights.' It would be more correct to say 'duties.' Every man will agree that in doing the job of a juryman, a witness, a telegraph clerk, we feel we are performing duties. And therefore it would be correct to say that women are seeking duties, and quite legitimately. And one can but sympathize with this desire to assist in the general labor of man."

"Quite so," said Alexey Alexandrovitch. "The question, I imagine, is simply whether they are fitted for such duties."[15]

Jury service, whether in czarist Russia or in the United States, can be quite intelligibly described both as a duty *and* as a right, though it is more likely to be described as the former by a harrassed and annoyed citizen grudgingly performing the service, and as the latter by the victim of discrimination who is excluded from the process. The same can be said for many other irksome chores in the "general labor of man."

Indeed *any* duty can be thought of also as a right. As we have seen, the statement of a duty trivially entails the statement of a "liberty," not a liberty in the usual sense that implies a choice but a liberty only in the sense made familiar by the jurisprudence textbooks, namely that of "no duty not to."[16] "Jones must do X" entails that "Jones may do X," and if Jones is to be guaranteed an opportunity to do what he must and may do, then others must not prevent him from doing it. If doing his duty happens also to be something from which Jones himself will benefit and Jones wants very much to do it, he will view his "liberty" or "permission" to do it, together with his guaranteed opportunity to do it, as goods that he can *claim* from others, and/or the state. Its character as claim is precisely what his liberty shares with the more customary (discretionary) rights and warrants his use of the term "right" in claiming it.

We have a choice between two ways of viewing the right to life, and whichever way we choose will have profound normative consequences. On the one hand, we can think of the right to life as a discretionary right analogous to many of the rights we have in the categories of liberty and property. My right to freedom of movement, for example, entitles me to travel where I wish or not to travel at all. It's entirely

15. Leo Tolstoy, *Anna Karenina* (New York, 1966), Part 4, chap. 10.
16. The textbook sense of "liberty" (derived from Hohfeld) would be less misleadingly called a "half-liberty." In ordinary speech, to be at liberty to do *x* is to have no duty in respect to *x*, that is (a) to be free of the duty not to do *x*, and (b) to be free of the duty to do *x*. To be free of a duty not to do *x* is to have only a half-liberty with respect to *x* if one should at the same time have a duty to do *x*. One is deprived, in that case, of the other "half-liberty" that would add up to full liberty, or discretion to decide whether to do *x* or not.

up to me. I have a right to go to Boston, but I can happily *waive* that right and go to Chicago, or I can stay at home if I prefer. When it comes to such general questions of my movement, I am the boss, or as Golding says, I reign sovereign over these aspects of my life.[17] Similarly, I have a right to all the money in my wallet and in my bank account. To say that it is *mine* or belongs to me is precisely to say that I can do with it as I please: spend it on food or clothing or amusement, or not spend it at all, or simply give it away. I have a right, of course to keep it, but that is a right I cheerfully *waive* when I donate it instead to a charity. On this model, my life, too, is mine; it belongs to me; I am sovereign over it; in respect to living or dying insofar as that rests within my power, I am the boss. I have a right, of course, to stay alive as long as I can, but I can *waive* that right, if I honestly and voluntarily choose to do so, and choose to die instead.

Alternatively, we can think of the right to life as a mandatory right analogous to the child's right to education, the criminal's right (on the Hegelian view) to punishment, or even the citizen's right to serve on juries. In that case, it can be viewed from one side as primarily a duty, something incumbent on us whatever our wishes about the matter may be. The right to life, so viewed, is a duty to stay alive as long as one can or, at least, a duty not to take one's own life or not to cooperate with others in its taking. Since life is generally an extremely important benefit to a person, indeed a condition of almost all other benefits, it is generally important to him that he be protected in his ability to exercise that duty. That protection takes the form of an enforced claim against all others to their noninterference, and that claim is his right to life seen from another vantage point. But, unlike discretionary rights, it can never be waived, and can be "exercised" in only one way. On this view, even if life is a "gift," it is a gift that cannot ever be declined or given away.

III. The Concept of an Inalienable Right

Rights are not mere abstract concepts; they are instruments and devices that can be used by their possessors to *do* things. A full theory of the nature of rights, therefore, would explain how they can be

17. Golding, "Towards a Theory of Human Rights," p. 547.

reserved, waived, renounced, transferred, sold; surrendered, forfeited, prescribed (cf. "imprescriptible"); annulled or made void, withdrawn, canceled; overruled, overridden, outbalanced; invaded, infringed, violated; recognized, enforced, vindicated, respected; possessed, enjoyed, exercised, stood upon, acted on, abused; acquired, inherited, purchased. Indeed some categories of rights are defined in terms of the uses to which they may or may not be put. An inalienable right, for example, is a right that may not be alienated. To understand what a right in this category is or would be, we must first understand what it would be like to alienate a right. On this question there has been a great deal of confusion for two centuries largely because of a failure to distinguish alienating from two other things from the list of things that can be done with rights, namely, forfeiting and annulling, and also a failure to distinguish between two possible interpretations of alienating, namely, waiving and relinquishing. I shall take up these notions in turn.

Alienating vs. Forfeiting

It was an important part of the classic doctrine of natural rights as expounded by Locke and Blackstone that some natural rights at least (certainly including the right to life) can be forfeited but not alienated. The distinction is roughly that between losing a right through one's fault or error, on the one hand, and voluntarily giving the right away, on the other. To forfeit, says Webster's, is "to lose or lose the right to, by some *error*, *fault*, *offense*, or *crime*; to alienate the right to possess *by some neglect or crime*; to have to pay as forfeit; as, to forfeit an estate by treason; to forfeit reputation" (emphasis added). A forfeitable right, therefore, cannot be an absolute one in our original sense, for it is not possessed unconditionally in all circumstances. Rather it is a right that one must qualify for by meeting certain conditions of proper conduct. As soon as one's conduct falls below the qualifying standards one loses the right, whether one likes it or not. Sometimes the loss is thought to occur instantly and naturally—for example, at the moment a homicidal aggressor puts another's life in jeopardy, his own life is forfeit to his threatened victim; at the moment a murderer kills his victim, he has ipso facto lost his own right to life against the state. In other cases, when the possessor of a forfeitable right misbehaves, he disqualifies himself for continued possession and becomes liable to the annulment of the right at a later time at the pleasure of the state—for example, a negligent motorist may be deprived of his driver's license in a proceeding that occurs a week after his misconduct. Since the forfeited right in all cases was originally understood to be conditional on the possessor's continued proper conduct, it is often said that disqualification is something he has brought upon himself, not of course as part of his explicit intention or motive in acting, but rather as the predictable and avoidable consequence of his wrongdoing. A forfeited right is not one that has been arbitrarily canceled or withdrawn, nor is it one that has been voluntarily relinquished or transferred. Rather it is thought to be one whose possessor has carelessly, stupidly, or recklessly allowed it to get away from him.

There is at least one striking paradox in the traditional view that the right to life can be forfeited (by the condemned murderer where capital punishment is permitted by law) but not voluntarily alienated. The would-be suicide can lose the right to life he no longer wants only by murdering someone else and thereby forfeiting the right that keeps him from his desired death. The inalienability of his right to life permits him to shed that unwanted life only by taking the life of someone else and thereby forfeiting it. Those who believe in the inalienability of the right to life, therefore, might well think twice before endorsing its forfeitability. A *nonforfeitable right* is one that a person cannot lose through his own blundering or wrongdoing; an *inalienable right* is one that a person cannot give away or dispense with through his own deliberate choice. Whenever the right in question can be thought of as burdensome baggage, it cannot be made inalienable *and* forfeitable without encouraging wrongdoing—the pursuit of relief through "error, fault, offense, or crime."

Alienating vs. Annulling

The major source of confusion in criticisms of the doctrine of inalienable rights over the last century or so might have been obviated, as B. A. Richards suggests,[18] by consulting a good dictionary. Many commentators have assumed uncritically that the founding fathers

18. B.A. Richards, "Inalienable Rights: Recent Criticism and Old Doctrine," *Philosophy and Phenomenological Research* 29 (1969): 398 n.

meant by an "inalienable right" one that could not be canceled or withdrawn by the state. In fact, natural rights theorists tended to use the word "indefeasible" for a right that cannot be taken away from its possessor by others, and most of them, as we have seen, following Richards, explicitly denied that the natural rights with which "all men are endowed by their Creator" are indefeasible in this sense. Webster's gives two senses of "inalienable": (1) "indefeasible: incapable of being annulled or made void," (2) "incapable of being alienated, surrendered, or transferred to another." Almost certainly, it was the second of these two senses that was intended by the founding fathers. Most eighteenth-century manifestoes and constitutions state or imply that the natural rights they invoke are subject to legitimate limitation. This implication, together with numerous statements in correspondence and philosophical essays that natural rights can be "abridged or modified in their exercise," strongly suggests that the founding fathers did not think of those rights as "indefeasible." An inalienable right, in the sense most likely intended by such early American writers as Paine and Jefferson is (in Webster's words) a right that "one cannot give away or dispose of even if one wishes." An indefeasible right, in contrast, is a right that "one cannot be deprived of without one's consent."

It is, of course, possible to hold that some rights are both inalienable and indefeasible, and perhaps this was the actual view of *some* of the founding fathers. But, putting the question of abridgement and annulment aside, there is no doubt that the distinctive and emphatic aspect of the doctrine of inalienability upon which almost all the founders agreed is that an inalienable right cannot be voluntarily given up or given away by its possessor. A very clear and typical statement of this doctrine and its supporting reasons, quoted by Richards, is that of Samuel Adams in "The Rights of Colonists." He says there that it would be

the greatest absurdity to suppose it in the power of one or any number of men at the entering into society, to renounce their essential natural rights, or the means of preserving those rights when the great end of civil government . . . is for the support, protection, and defence of those very rights: the principal of which . . . are life, liberty, and property. If men through fear, fraud, or mistake, should in terms renounce and give up any essential natural right, the eternal law of reason . . . would absolutely vacate such renunciation; the right to freedom being the gift of God Almighty, it is not in the power of Man to alienate this gift, and voluntarily become a slave.[19]

Several arguments are only vaguely suggested in the passage quoted, but there is nothing vague about Adams' conclusion. Adams finds it irrational for anyone to renounce a natural right and implies that such renunciations must be prompted by "fear, fraud, or mistake," thereby failing to be wholly voluntary. But even if such a renunciation were somehow made without mistake, fraud, or reason-numbing fear, it would be invalid on the grounds that a "gift" from an all-powerful Creator cannot, in the very nature of things, be refused or relinquished. Whatever we are to make of these arguments, there can be no doubt what conclusion they are meant to support: the right to life, like the other natural rights, "cannot be given away or disposed of, even if one wishes."

Waiving vs. Relinquishing

Failure to distinguish between waiving exercise of a right that one continues to possess and relinquishing one's very possession of the right can leave the doctrine of inalienability ambiguous and uncertain in its application to the problems of suicide and voluntary euthanasia. What exactly is it that cannot be alienated when one has an inalienable right to X—X itself or the right to X? If it is X itself that cannot be voluntarily alienated (abandoned, transferred, sold, and so on) then the right to X is a mandatory right, and one has a duty to do X or continue in possession of X. In that case, one is not at liberty to waive his right to X in some circumstances while insisting on it in others, at his discretion. If the right to life is inalienable in this strong sense, then we have a duty to continue to live and forbear suicide that we cannot waive, for it would not merely be our right to life that is inalienable but our life itself. On the other hand, if it is the right which is inalienable, as opposed to that to which it is a right, then it

19. Quoted by Richards, p. 398 n.

might yet be true that the right in question is a discretionary right (as is my right to move to Chicago or to read Joyce's *Ulysses* or to keep strangers off my land) which I can exercise or decline to exercise as I choose. To *waive* my discretionary right is to exercise my power to release others from correlative duties to me, to desist from claiming my right against them, as when I waive my right to exclusive enjoyment of my land by inviting in a stranger. To be sure, in other cases, such as moving to Chicago or reading *Ulysses*, failure to exercise a right is not called "waiving" it since the obligations of other parties are not affected in the appropriate way. But what is important for our present purposes is what "declining to exercise" and "waiving" have in common, namely the protected discretion to act or not as one chooses. It does not follow from the inalienability of the *right* to life, that I may not decline to exercise it positively or that I cannot waive it (by releasing others from their duties not to kill me or let me die) if I choose. If I decline to exercise the right in a positive way or else waive it, then it is my *life* that I alienate, not my right to life.

It will be useful at this point to illustrate this distinction by using it to generate two possible interpretations of the "inalienability" of the natural rights to property and liberty, as well as to life. Consider first the *right to* property. What would it be like to waive or decline to exercise the right, while keeping possession of it, that is, "reserving" it? One might sell all one's goods and then give away the money, and live thenceforth by begging. That would be to exercise one's right to property, interpreted as a discretionary right, in a negative way. So interpreted, one has a right to acquire property or not to acquire it, to "take it or leave it," as one chooses, just as one has a right to acquire as little or as much as one can. When I give all of my property away, I have not abandoned the discretionary right to acquire (or re-acquire) property; rather I have chosen to exercise that right in a particular, eccentric, way.

It is less clear what would be involved in relinquishing the right to property itself. Here we must imagine a constitutional order and a legal system in which the right to property itself is alienable. Perhaps under such a regime one could formally renounce one's right to acquire property in a legally binding way, thus relinquishing the right irrevocably (unless the system also provided some legal procedure for re-acquiring renounced rights). If one were thus permitted to relinquish the right permanently, one could possess objects and occupy places but never *own* them. One would be a member of a special lower order of citizenship in that respect, or perhaps a permanent member of a mendicant religious order whose vow of permanent poverty is now enforced by the state at his own original request.

Waiving one's right to all *liberty* for a period while continuing to possess the discretionary right to liberty is illustrated by a story that is somewhat more fanciful but no less coherent than the parallel story about the right to property. One might lock oneself in a room and throw away the key, having arranged to have one's food put in through the transom, and one's garbage hauled out daily until further notice. As a consequence, one would no longer be at liberty to come and go as one pleases except within the narrow and quite minimal confines of a small cell-like room. If contact with delivery and disposal men is scheduled daily at 9:00 A.M. and one finally decides to terminate the arrangement one morning at 10:00, then one will still have to go twenty-three more hours without one's natural liberty. But, in virtue of one's continued possession of the right to liberty throughout the period during which it is voluntarily waived, liberty itself can be re-acquired in time.

In contrast, if the legal system permitted one to alienate the right to liberty itself, and to do so permanently and irrevocably, then one's future enjoyment of liberty would be sporadic, limited, and entirely subject to the pleasure of other parties. The story illustrating this possibility is that of a person who formally contracts to become the permanent chattel-slave of another, in exchange for some initial "consideration," perhaps one million dollars to be paid in advance to a beneficiary or favorite cause of the contractor. Once he becomes a slave he is no longer free to come and go as *he* chooses, but only as commanded or permitted by his master.

When we turn from property and liberty to life, we discover an apparent asymmetry. Until now, we have been able to distinguish without much difficulty between alienating X and alienating the right to X and to give plausible illustrations of each. But where X stands for life there is an apparent difficulty. In the other cases, I could give up X, at least for a time, without relinquishing the right to X. I could give away my money, or throw away the key to my locked room without resigning my right to re-acquire property or liberty. But I cannot destroy my life for a period of time while maintaining my discretionary right to re-acquire life whenever I so choose. Thus, an illustration of the waiver or nonexercise of a maintained right to life cannot take the form of a story of a person who deliberately has himself killed. Nevertheless, despite this important difference from the other cases, the distinction between waiving and relinquishing can be applied, albeit in a distinctive way, to the right to life too.

An illustration of a temporary waiver of the right to life was suggested to me by Don E. Scheid. Imagine a community that has celebrated from time immemorial an annual spring rite. One of the traditional rituals is a kind of sporting contest in which all of the males of a certain age are encouraged, but not required, to participate. All the "players" are armed with knives, clubs, bows, and arrows, and then turned loose in a large forest. For an hour every man is both hunter and prey. For that period of time the normal right to life is suspended for all the voluntary participants. In effect, therefore, each has *waived* the protection of that right for a fixed period of time, with no possibility of repossessing it until the time is up and the game is over. Each player thus releases all of the other players from their normal obligation not to kill him. The object of the game is twofold: to stay alive oneself until the game is over and to kill as many of the others as one can. This is a fanciful but coherent illustration of a set of rules that confer on everyone a discretionary right to life and also the power to waive that right (thus exercising it negatively) while the right continues to remain in one's possession.

The example of the formal renunciation and irrevocable relinquishment of the right to life is closely similar to the corresponding cases of permanent abandonment of the rights to property and liberty. Now we must imagine a legal system so permissive that it allows one formally to contract with another, again for a sizable consideration paid to third parties in advance, to put one's life—one's continued existence—in the other's legal power. I consent, in this bizarre example, to the other's irrevocable right to kill me if or whenever *he* decides to do so. He may have no other legal control over me except that derived from the power of his threat to exercise his right to kill.

Technically, I am not his chattel or slave and am at liberty to accumulate property and move about at will, as long, of course, as I stay alive. I *might* stay alive indefinitely, even to the point of my natural death, provided my legitimate killer decides to be benevolent. But if he chooses to exercise his contractual right in another fashion, he may wipe me out, as he may swat a fly or squash a bug, since I have no more claim on his forbearance than does an insect.

The sense in which a right is "waived" in the example of the spring rite is not *very* different from that in which rights are "renounced" in the examples using slavery and a contract to kill. The difference is best understood as one of degree. In the contract examples, the right in question is renounced permanently and irrevocably; the renouncer can never get his right back simply by changing his mind. In the spring-rite example, the right is in effect irrevocably renounced for *a fixed period of time*; no change of mind during that period can restore the right to its original owner. But after the expiration of that interval, the right can be repossessed. "Waiving" a right in a second, weaker but more natural, sense is to give it up provisionally without relinquishing the right to change one's mind *at any point* and thereby nullify the transaction. "Waiving the right to life" by means of a "living will" would be waiving in this sense. In short, there are two senses of "waiving": a stronger sense, which is actually short-term renunciation, and a more familiar weak sense in which waiving is inherently revocable. Voluntary euthanasia involves waiving in the latter sense; the spring rite involves waiving in the former; the contract to kill involves permanently irrevocable "waiving," which is the same thing as unconditional nullification, or renunciation.

IV. A RIGHT TO DIE? THREE VIEWS

How could a person have a right to terminate his own life (by his own hand or the hand of another) if his right to life is inalienable? It would probably be wise here to treat suicide as a special case that should be put aside to enable us to focus more narrowly on voluntary euthanasia. That is because suicide directly raises an additional philosophical perplexity, the puzzle of reflexive moral relations. If it is conceptually possible to violate one's own right to life by committing suicide, it must be the case that one's right to life is a claim addressed inter alia to oneself. In that case, I could have a duty *to myself* not to kill myself from which I cannot release myself, a situation many writers, from Aristotle on, have found incoherent or paradoxical. The paradox is not mitigated simply by thinking of the right to life as a mandatory right. I might well have a mandatory right to life—that is, a *duty* not to kill myself—which is owed to other people. In that case the involved claims are addressed not to myself but to others, claims to provide me with the opportunity to live and not to interfere with my discharge of my duty to live. No paradox arises in that case because no claim is self-addressed. Not all proposed mandatory rights are non-controversially coherent and intelligible, but only those that are asso- ,ciated with duties which, being owed to others, escape the problem of reflexive moral relations.

Most people in normal circumstances do have a duty not to kill themselves that is derived from the rights of other people who rely or depend on them. That duty can be thought of as a mandatory right because in the circumstances in question, its discharge also happens to be importantly beneficial to the person who possesses it. Moreover, that person can *claim* the associated half-liberties necessary for its exercise. But it is not a paradoxical mandatory right, because its claims are addressed to others (not to interfere), and the duty at its core is owed to others. In these circumstances of interpersonal reli- ance, one's general right to life, even if it is discretionary and absolute in its own domain, is subject to "territorial" limitation. One's own personal autonomy ends where the rights of others begin, just as national sovereignty comes to a limit at the boundaries of another nation's territory. My life may be my property, but there are limits to the uses to which I can put anything I own, and I may not destroy what is mine if I thereby destroy or seriously harm what does not belong to me. So some suicides may violate the rights of *other* persons, though equally certainly some suicides do not.

But how could my suicide violate my *own* right to life? Is that right a claim against myself as well as against others? Do I treat myself unjustly if I deliberately end my life for what seem to me the best

reasons?[20] Am I my own victim in that case? Do I have a moral grievance against myself? Is suicide just another case of murder? Am I
really two persons for the purposes of moral judgment, one an evil
wrong-doer and the other the wronged victim of the first's evil deed?
Can one of me be blamed or punished without blaming or punishing
the other? Perhaps these questions make the head reel because they
raise interestingly novel moral possibilities. On the other hand, their
paradoxes may derive, as the predominant philosophical tradition
maintains, from the conceptual violence they do to the integrity of
the self and the way we understand the concept of a right.

In either case we would be well advised to confine our attention to
voluntary euthanasia and ask whether a person who accedes to an
ailing friend's urgent and deliberate request by painlessly killing him
or letting him die, has violated that person's inalienable right to life.
Here at least is a question that is conceptually open and difficult. The
distinctions explained above between discretionary and mandatory
rights, indefeasible and inalienable rights, and between waiving and
relinquishing rights will enable us to formulate three possible positions. It will then be clear, I hope, which of the three can plausibly be
attributed to the founding fathers.

The Paternalist

According to the first possible view, the right to life is a nonwaivable,
mandatory right. On this view there is no right to die but only a right
to live. Since there is no morally permitted alternative to the one prescribed path, following it is a duty, like the duty of children to attend
school and the duty of convicted felons to undergo punishment. But
since continued life itself is a benefit in all circumstances whatever
the person whose life it is may think about it, we may with propriety

20. St. Thomas Aquinas grants the point, on the authority of Aristotle, that
nobody can commit an injustice to himself, even by committing suicide. The
sinfulness of suicide, according to Aquinas, consists not in the fact that one
violates one's own rights (which Aquinas finds incoherent) but rather in that
(a) the suicide violates God's rights just as in killing a slave one violates the
rights of the slave's master; (b) the suicide violates his community's rights by
depriving it of one of its "parts"; (c) the suicide acts against the *charity* (not
the justice) that a person should have towards himself. Aquinas therefore would
agree that the suicide, sinful though he may be, does not violate his own "right
to life." See *Summa Theologica,* vol. II, Question 64, A5.

refer to it as a right. In this respect, too, the right to life is similar to the right to education and the right to punishment (as understood by Hegelians). The "right to life" is essentially a duty, but expressible in the language of rights because the derivative claims against others that they save or not kill one are *necessarily* beneficial—goods that one could not rationally forswear. The right therefore must always be "exercised" and can never be "waived." Anyone who could wish to waive it must simply be ignorant of what is good for him.

The Founding Fathers

The second position differs sharply from the first in that it takes the right to life to be a discretionary, not a mandatory right. In this respect that right is exactly like the most treasured specimens in the "right to liberty" and "right to property" categories. Just as we have rights to come or go as we choose, to read or not read, to speak or not speak, to worship or not worship, to buy, sell, or sit tight, as we please, so we have a right, within the boundaries of our own autonomy, to live or die, as we choose. The right to die is simply the other side of the coin of the right to live. The basic right underlying each is the right to be one's own master, to dispose of one's own lot as one chooses, subject of course to the limits imposed by the like rights of others. Just as my right to live imposes a duty on others not to kill me, so my right to die, which it entails, imposes a duty on others not to prevent me from implementing my choice of death, except for the purpose of determining whether that choice is genuinely voluntary, hence truly mine. When I choose to die by my own hand, I insist upon my claim to the noninterference of others. When I am unable to terminate my own life, I *waive* my right to live in exercising my right to die, which is one and the same thing as releasing at least one other person from his duty not to kill me. In exercising my own choice in these matters, I am not renouncing, abjuring, forswearing, resigning, or relinquishing my right to life; quite the contrary, I am *acting* on that right by exercising it one way or the other. I cannot relinquish or effectively renounce the right, for that would be to alienate what is not properly alienable. To alienate the right would be to abandon my discretion; to waive the right is to exercise that discretion. The right itself, as opposed to that to which I have the right, is inalienable.

The state can properly prohibit such sanguinary frolics as the spring rite described above without annulling the discretionary right to life, just as the state may limit the right to property by levying taxes, or the right to liberty by requiring passports or imposing speed limits. To limit discretion in the public interest is not to cancel it or withdraw it. The spring rite is forbidden, not because our lives are not our own to risk (what is more risky than mountain climbing or car racing?), but rather because: (a) it cannot be in the public interest to permit widespread carnage, to deprive the population of a substantial portion of its most vital youthful members, and leave large numbers of dependent widows and orphans and heartbroken friends and relations; and (b) the "voluntariness" of the participation in such a ritual, like that of the private duel to death, must be suspect, given the pressure of public opinion, the liability to disgrace by nonparticipation, and the perceived inequality of skills among the participants. These are reasons enough for a legal prohibition even in a community that recognizes an indefeasible discretionary right to life (and death).

The Extreme Antipaternalist

The third position springs from a profound and understandable aversion to the smug paternalism of the first view. Like the second view, it interprets the right to life as a discretionary right which we may exercise as we please within the limits imposed by the like rights of others and the public interest. So far, I suspect, Paine, Adams, and Jefferson would be in solid agreement, since the natural rights emphasized in their rhetoric and later incorporated in our Constitution were, for the most part, protected options, and these writers made constant appeal to personal autonomy in their arguments about particular political issues. But this third view goes well beyond anything the fathers contemplated, since it holds that not only is life alienable; the discretionary right to life is alienable too. This view, of course, cannot be reconciled with the explicit affirmations of inalienability made in most of the leading documents of the revolutionary period, thus it cannot be attributed to the founding fathers. But it would be a mistake to dismiss it too quickly, for paternalism is a hard doctrine to compromise with, and it rejects paternalism *totally*. According to this third view, a free and autonomous person can renounce and relinquish any right, *provided only that his choice is fully informed, well considered, and uncoerced*, that is to say, *fully voluntary*. It may well be, as I have argued elsewhere, that there is no practicable and reliable way of discovering whether a choice to abjure a natural right is fully voluntary.[21] The evidence of voluntariness which we can acquire may never be sufficiently strong to override the natural presumption that no one in his right mind, fully informed, would sell himself into permanent poverty or slavery or sell his discretionary right to life. On that ground the state might always refuse to sanction requests from citizens that they be permitted to alienate the right to life. But that ground is quite consistent with the acknowledgment that even the natural right to life is alienable *in principle*, though not in fact. At least such a consistent antipaternalistic strategy would keep us from resorting, like Sam Adams, to the peculiar idea of a "gift" that cannot be declined, given away, or returned, and would enable us to avoid the even more peculiar notion that the right to life of an autonomous person is not properly his own at all, but rather the property of his creator.

Whatever judgment we make of the third position, however, will be consistent with the primary theses of this essay: that the inalienable right to life can be interpreted in such a way that it is not infringed by voluntary euthanasia; that that interpretation (the second position above) is coherent and reasonably plausible; and that it is very likely the account that best renders the actual intentions of Jefferson and the other founding fathers.

21. See the discussion in Joel Feinberg, "Legal Paternalism," *Canadian Journal of Philosophy* 1 (1971): 105-124.

PHILIPPA FOOT   Euthanasia

The widely used *Shorter Oxford English Dictionary* gives three meanings for the word "euthanasia": the first, "a quiet and easy death"; the
second, "the means of procuring this"; and the third, "the action of
inducing a quiet and easy death." It is a curious fact that no one of the
three gives an adequate definition of the word as it is usually understood. For "euthanasia" means much more than a quiet and easy
death, or the means of procuring it, or the action of inducing it. The
definition specifies only the manner of the death, and if this were all
that was implied a murderer, careful to drug his victim, could claim
that his act was an act of euthanasia. We find this ridiculous because
we take it for granted that in euthanasia it is death itself, not just the
manner of death, that must be kind to the one who dies.

To see how important it is that "euthanasia" should not be used as
the dictionary definition allows it to be used, merely to signifiy that a
death was quiet and easy, one has only to remember that Hitler's
"euthanasia" program traded on this ambiguity. Under this program,
planned before the War but brought into full operation by a decree
of 1 September 1939, some 275,000 people were gassed in centers
which were to be a model for those in which Jews were later exter-
minated. Anyone in a state institution could be sent to the gas cham-
bers if it was considered that he could not be "rehabilitated" for useful
work. As Dr. Leo Alexander reports, relying on the testimony of a

© 1977 by Philippa Foot, reprinted by permission.

I would like to thank Derek Parfit and the Editors of *Philosophy & Public
Affairs* for their very helpful comments.

neuropathologist who received 500 brains from one of the killing centers,

> In Germany the exterminations included the mentally defective, psychotics (particularly schizophrenics), epileptics and patients suffering from infirmities of old age and from various organic neurological disorders such as infantile paralysis, Parkinsonism, multiple sclerosis and brain tumors. . . . In truth, all those unable to work and considered nonrehabilitable were killed.[1]

These people were killed because they were "useless" and "a burden on society"; only the manner of their deaths could be thought of as relatively easy and quiet.

Let us insist, then, that when we talk about euthanasia we are talking about a death understood as a good or happy event for the one who dies. This stipulation follows etymology, but is itself not exactly in line with current usage, which would be captured by the condition that the death should *not* be an evil rather than that it *should* be a good. That this is how people talk is shown by the fact that the case of Karen Ann Quinlan and others in a state of permanent coma is often discussed under the heading of "euthanasia." Perhaps it is not too late to object to the use of the word "euthanasia" in this sense. Apart from the break with the Greek origins of the word there are other unfortunate aspects of this extension of the term. For if we say that the death must be supposed to be a good to the subject we can also specify that it shall be for his sake that an act of euthanasia is performed. If we say merely that death shall not be an evil to him, we cannot stipulate that benefiting him shall be the motive where euthanasia is in question. Given the importance of the question, For whose sake are we acting? it is good to have a definition of euthanasia which brings under this heading only cases of opting for death for the sake of the one who dies. Perhaps what is most important is to say either that euthanasia is to be for the good of the subject or at least that death is to be no evil to him, thus refusing to talk Hitler's language. However, in this paper it is the first condition that will be understood, with the additional proviso that by an act of euthanasia we mean one

---

1. Leo Alexander, "Medical Science under Dictatorship," *New England Journal of Medicine*, 14 July 1949, p. 40.

of inducing or otherwise opting for death for the sake of the one who is to die.

A few lesser points need to be cleared up. In the first place it must be said that the word "act" is not to be taken to exclude omission: we shall speak of an act of euthanasia when someone is deliberately allowed to die, for his own good, and not only when positive measures are taken to see that he does. The very general idea we want is that of a choice of action or inaction directed at another man's death and causally effective in the sense that, in conjunction with actual circumstances, it is a sufficient condition of death. Of complications such as overdetermination, it will not be necessary to speak.

A second, and definitely minor, point about the definition of an act of euthanasia concerns the question of fact versus belief. It has already been implied that one who performs an act of euthanasia thinks that death will be merciful for the subject since we have said that it is on account of this thought that the act is done. But is it enough that he acts with this thought, or must things actually be as he thinks them to be? If one man kills another, or allows him to die, thinking that he is in the last stages of a terrible disease, though in fact he could have been cured, is this an act of euthanasia or not? Nothing much seems to hang on our decision about this. The same condition has got to enter into the definition whether as an element in reality or only as an element in the agent's belief. And however we define an act of euthanasia culpability or justifiability will be the same: if a man acts through ignorance his ignorance may be culpable or it may not.[2]

These are relatively easy problems to solve, but one that is dauntingly difficult has been passed over in this discussion of the definition, and must now be faced. It is easy to say, as if this raised no problems, that an act of euthanasia is by definition one aiming at the *good* of the one whose death is in question, and that it is *for his sake* that his death is desired. But how is this to be explained? Presumably we are thinking of some evil already with him or to come on him if he continues to live, and death is thought of as a release from this evil. But this

2. For a discussion of culpable and nonculpable ignorance see Thomas Aquinas, *Summa Theologica*, First Part of the Second Part, Question 6, article 8, and Question 19, articles 5 and 6.

cannot be enough. Most people's lives contain evils such as grief or pain, but we do not therefore think that death would be a blessing to them. On the contrary life is generally supposed to be a good even for someone who is unusually unhappy or frustrated. How is it that one can ever wish for death for the sake of the one who is to die? This difficult question is central to the discussion of euthanasia, and we shall literally not know what we are talking about if we ask whether acts of euthanasia defined as we have defined them are ever morally permissible without first understanding better the reason for saying that life is a good, and the possibility that it is not always so.

If a man should save my life he would be my benefactor. In normal circumstances this is plainly true; but does one always benefit another in saving his life? It seems certain that he does not. Suppose, for instance, that a man were being tortured to death and was given a drug that lengthened his sufferings; this would not be a benefit but the reverse. Or suppose that in a ghetto in Nazi Germany a doctor saved the life of someone threatened by disease, but that the man once cured was transported to an extermination camp; the doctor might wish for the sake of the patient that he had died of the disease. Nor would a longer stretch of life always be a benefit to the person who was given it. Comparing Hitler's camps with those of Stalin, Dmitri Panin observes that in the latter the method of extermination was made worse by agonies that could stretch out over months.

> Death from a bullet would have been bliss compared with what many millions had to endure while dying of hunger. The kind of death to which they were condemned has nothing to equal it in treachery and sadism.[3]

These examples show that to save or prolong a man's life is not always to do him a service: it may be better for him if he dies earlier rather than later. It must therefore be agreed that while life is normally a benefit to the one who has it, this is not always so.

The judgment is often fairly easy to make—that life is or is not a good to someone—but the basis for it is very hard to find. When life is said to be a benefit or a good, on what grounds is the assertion made? The difficulty is underestimated if it is supposed that the problem

---

3. Dmitri Panin, *The Notebooks of Sologdin* (London. 1976), pp. 66–67.

arises from the fact that one who is dead has nothing, so that the good someone gets from being alive cannot be compared with the amount he would otherwise have had. For why should this particular comparison be necessary? Surely it would be enough if one could say whether or not someone whose life was prolonged had more good than evil in the extra stretch of time. Such estimates are not always possible, but frequently they are; we say, for example, "He was very happy in those last years," or, "He had little but unhappiness then." If the balance of good and evil determined whether life was a good to someone we would expect to find a correlation in the judgments. In fact, of course, we find nothing of the kind. First, a man who has no doubt that existence is a good to him may have no idea about the balance of happiness and unhappiness in his life, or of any other positive and negative factors that may be suggested. So the supposed criteria are not always operating where the judgment is made. And secondly the application of the criteria gives an answer that is often wrong. Many people have more evil than good in their lives; we do not, however, conclude that we would do these people no service by rescuing them from death.

To get around this last difficulty Thomas Nagel has suggested that experience itself is a good which must be brought in to balance accounts.

> . . . life is worth living even when the bad elements of experience are plentiful, and the good ones too meager to outweigh the bad ones on their own. The additional positive weight is supplied by experience itself, rather than by any of its contents.[4]

This seems implausible because if experience itself is a good it must be so even when what we experience is wholly bad, as in being tortured to death. How should one decide how much to count for this experiencing; and why count anything at all?

Others have tried to solve the problem by arguing that it is a man's desire for life that makes us call life a good: if he wants to live then anyone who prolongs his life does him a benefit. Yet someone may cling to life where we would say confidently that it would be better

---

4. Thomas Nagel, "Death," in James Rachels, ed., *Moral Problems* (New York, 1971), p. 362.

for him if he died, and he may admit it too. Speaking of those same conditions in which, as he said, a bullet would have been merciful, Panin writes,

> I should like to pass on my observations concerning the absence of suicides under the extremely severe conditions of our concentration camps. The more that life became desperate, the more a prisoner seemed determined to hold onto it.[5]

One might try to explain this by saying that hope was the ground of this wish to survive for further days and months in the camp. But there is nothing unintelligible in the idea that a man might cling to life though he knew those facts about his future which would make any charitable man wish that he might die.

The problem remains, and it is hard to know where to look for a solution. Is there a conceptual connection between *life* and *good*? Because life is not always a good we are apt to reject this idea, and to think that it must be a contingent fact that life is usually a good, as it is a contingent matter that legacies are usually a benefit, if they are. Yet it seems not to be a contingent matter that to save someone's life is ordinarily to benefit him. The problem is to find where the conceptual connection lies.

It may be good tactics to forget for a time that it is euthanasia we are discussing and to see how *life* and *good* are connected in the case of living beings other than men. Even plants have things done to them that are harmful or beneficial, and what does them good must be related in some way to their living and dying. Let us therefore consider plants and animals, and then come back to human beings. At least we shall get away from the temptation to think that the connection between life and benefit must everywhere be a matter of happiness and unhappiness or of pleasure and pain; the idea being absurd in the case of animals and impossible even to formulate for plants.

In case anyone thinks that the concept of the beneficial applies only in a secondary or analogical way to plants, he should be reminded that we speak quite straightforwardly in saying, for instance, that a certain amount of sunlight is beneficial to most plants. What is in

5. Panin, *Sologdin*, p. 85.

question here is the habitat in which plants of particular species flourish, but we can also talk, in a slightly different way, of what does them good, where there is some suggestion of improvement or remedy. What has the beneficial to do with sustaining life? It is tempting to answer, "everything," thinking that a healthy condition just is the one apt to secure survival. In fact, however, what is beneficial to a plant may have to do with reproduction rather than the survival of the individual member of the species. Nevertheless there is a plain connection between the beneficial and the life-sustaining even for the individual plant; if something makes it better able to survive in conditions normal for that species it is ipso facto good for it. We need go no further, and could go no further, in explaining why a certain environment or treatment is good for a plant than to show how it helps this plant to survive.[6]

This connection between the life-sustaining and the beneficial is reasonably unproblematic, and there is nothing fanciful or zoomorphic in speaking of benefiting or doing good to plants. A connection with its survival can make something beneficial to a plant. But this is not, of course, to say that we count life as a good to a plant. We may save its life by giving it what is beneficial; we do not benefit it by saving its life.

A more ramified concept of benefit is used in speaking of animal life. New things can be said, such as that an animal is better or worse off for something that happened, or that it was a good or bad thing for it that it did happen. And new things count as benefit. In the first place, there is comfort, which often is, but need not be, related to health. When loosening a collar which is too tight for a dog we can say, "That will be better for it." So we see that the words "better for it" have two different meanings which we mark when necessary by a difference of emphasis, saying "better *for* it" when health is involved. And secondly an animal can be benefited by having its life saved. "Could you do anything for it?" can be answered by, "Yes, I managed to save its life." Sometimes we may understand this, just as we would

6. Yet some detail needs to be filled in to explain why we should not say that a scarecrow is beneficial to the plants it protects. Perhaps what is beneficial must either be a feature of the plant itself, such as protective prickles, or else must work on the plant directly, such as a line of trees which give it shade.

for a plant, to mean that we had checked some disease. But we can also do something for an animal by scaring away its predator. If we do this, it is a good thing for the animal that we did, unless of course it immediately meets a more unpleasant end by some other means. Similarly, on the bad side, an animal may be worse off for our intervention, and this not because it pines or suffers but simply because it gets killed.

The problem that vexes us when we think about euthanasia comes on the scene at this point. For if we can do something for an animal—can benefit it—by relieving its suffering but also by saving its life, where does the greater benefit come when only death will end pain? It seemed that life was a good in its own right; yet pain seemed to be an evil with equal status and could therefore make life not a good after all. Is it only life without pain that is a good when animals are concerned? This does not seem a crazy suggestion when we are thinking of animals, since unlike human beings they do not have suffering as part of their normal life. But it is perhaps the idea of ordinary life that matters here. We would not say that we had done anything for an animal if we had merely kept it alive, either in an unconscious state or in a condition where, though conscious, it was unable to operate in an ordinary way; and the fact is that animals in severe and continuous pain simply do not operate normally. So we do not, on the whole, have the option of doing the animal good by saving its life though the life would be a life of pain. No doubt there are borderline cases, but that is no problem. We are not trying to make new judgments possible, but rather to find the principle of the ones we do make.

When we reach human life the problems seem even more troublesome. For now we must take quite new things into account, such as the subject's own view of his life. It is arguable that this places extra constraints on the solution: might it not be counted as a necessary condition of life's being a good to a man that he should see it as such? Is there not some difficulty about the idea that a benefit might be done to him by the saving or prolonging of his life even though he himself wished for death? Of course he might have a quite mistaken view of his own prospects, but let us ignore this and think only of cases where it is life as he knows it that is in question. Can we think that the prolonging of this life would be a benefit to him even though he would rather have it end than continue? It seems that this cannot be ruled out. That there is no simple incompatibility between life as a good and the wish for death is shown by the possibility that a man should wish himself dead, not for his own sake, but for the sake of someone else. And if we try to amend the thesis to say that life cannot be a good to one who wishes *for his own sake* that he should die, we find the crucial concept slipping through our fingers. As Bishop Butler pointed out long ago not all ends are either benevolent or self-interested. Does a man wish for death for his own sake in the relevant sense if, for instance, he wishes to revenge himself on another by his death. Or what if he is proud and refuses to stomach dependence or incapacity even though there are many good things left in life for him? The truth seems to be that the wish for death is sometimes compatible with life's being a good and sometimes not, which is possible because the description "wishing for death" is one covering diverse states of mind from that of the determined suicide, pathologically depressed, to that of one who is surprised to find that the thought of a fatal accident is viewed with relief. On the one hand, a man may see his life as a burden but go about his business in a more or less ordinary way; on the other hand, the wish for death may take the form of a rejection of everything that is in life, as it does in severe depression. It seems reasonable to say that life is not a good to one permanently in the latter state, and we must return to this topic later on.

When are we to say that life is a good or a benefit to a man? The dilemma that faces us is this. If we say that life as such is a good we find ourselves refuted by the examples given at the beginning of this discussion. We therefore incline to think that it is as bringing good things that life is a good, where it is a good. But if life is a good only because it is the condition of good things why is it not equally an evil when it brings bad things? And how can it be a good even when it brings more evil than good?

It should be noted that the problem has here been formulated in terms of the balance of good and evil, not that of happiness and unhappiness, and that it is not to be solved by the denial (which may be reasonable enough) that unhappiness is the only evil or happiness the only good. In this paper no view has been expressed about the nature of goods other than life itself. The point is that on any view of the goods and evils that life can contain, it seems that a life with more evil than good could still itself be a good.

It may be useful to review the judgments with which our theory must square. Do we think that life can be a good to one who suffers a lot of pain? Clearly we do. What about severely handicapped people; can life be a good to them? Clearly it can be, for even if someone is almost completely paralyzed, perhaps living in an iron lung, perhaps able to move things only by means of a tube held between his lips, we do not rule him out of order if he says that some benefactor saved his life. Nor is it different with mental handicap. There are many fairly severely handicapped people—such as those with Down's Syndrome (Mongolism)—for whom a simple affectionate life is possible. What about senility? Does this break the normal connection between life and good? Here we must surely distinguish between forms of senility. Some forms leave a life which we count someone as better off having than not having, so that a doctor who prolonged it would benefit the person concerned. With some kinds of senility this is however no longer true. There are some in geriatric wards who are barely conscious, though they can move a little and swallow food put into their mouths. To prolong such a state, whether in the old or in the very severely mentally handicapped is not to do them a service or confer a benefit. But of course it need not be the reverse: only if there is suffering would one wish for the sake of the patient that he should die.

It seems, therefore, that merely being alive even without suffering is not a good, and that we must make a distinction similar to that which we made when animals were our topic. But how is the line to be drawn in the case of men? What is to count as ordinary human life in the relevant sense? If it were only the very senile or very ill who were to be said not to have this life it might seem right to describe it in terms of *operation*. But it will be hard to find the sense in which the men described by Panin were not operating, given that they dragged themselves out to the forest to work. What is it about the life that the prisoners were living that makes us put it on the other side of the dividing line from that of some severely ill or suffering patients, and from most of the physically or mentally handicapped?

It is not that they were in captivity, for life in captivity can certainly be a good. Nor is it merely the unusual nature of their life. In some ways the prisoners were living more as other men do than the patient in an iron lung.

The suggested solution to the problem is, then, that there is a certain conceptual connection between *life* and *good* in the case of human beings as in that of animals and even plants. Here, as there, however, it is not the mere state of being alive that can determine, or itself count as, a good, but rather life coming up to some standard of normality. It was argued that it is as part of ordinary life that the elements of good that a man may have are relevant to the question of whether saving his life counts as benefiting him. Ordinary human lives, even very hard lives, contain a minimum of basic goods, but when these are absent the idea of life is no longer linked to that of good. And since it is in this way that the elements of good contained in a man's life are relevant to the question of whether he is benefited if his life is preserved, there is no reason why it should be the balance of good and evil that counts.

It should be added that evils are relevant in one way when, as in the examples discussed above, they destroy the possibility of ordinary goods, but in a different way when they invade a life from which the goods are already absent for a different reason. So, for instance, the connection between *life* and *good* may be broken because consciousness has sunk to a very low level, as in extreme senility or severe brain damage. In itself this kind of life seems to be neither good nor evil, but if suffering sets in one would hope for a speedy end.

The idea we need seems to be that of life which is ordinary human life in the following respect—that it contains a minimum of basic human goods. What is ordinary in human life—even in very hard lives —is that a man is not driven to work far beyond his capacity; that he has the support of a family or community; that he can more or less satisfy his hunger; that he has hopes for the future; that he can lie down to rest at night. Such things were denied to the men in the Vyatlag camps described by Panin; not even rest at night was allowed them when they were tormented by bed-bugs, by noise and stench, and by routines such as body-searches and bath-parades—arranged for the night time so that work norms would not be reduced. Disease too can so take over a man's life that the normal human goods disappear. When a patient is so overwhelmed by pain or nausea that he cannot eat with pleasure, if he can eat at all, and is out of the reach of even the most loving voice, he no longer has ordinary human life in the sense in which the words are used here. And we may now pick up a thread from an earlier part of the discussion by remarking that crippling depression can destroy the enjoyment of ordinary goods as effectively as external circumstances can remove them.

This, admittedly inadequate, discussion of the sense in which life is normally a good, and of the reasons why it may not be so in some particular case, completes the account of what euthanasia is here taken to be. An act of euthanasia, whether literally act or rather omission, is attributed to an agent who opts for the death of another because in his case life seems to be an evil rather than a good. The question now to be asked is whether acts of euthanasia are ever justifiable. But there are two topics here rather than one. For it is one thing to say that some acts of euthanasia considered only in themselves and their results are morally unobjectionable, and another to say that it would be all right to legalize them. Perhaps the practice of euthanasia would allow too many abuses, and perhaps there would be too many mistakes. Moreover the practice might have very important and highly undesirable side effects, because it is unlikely that we could change our principles about the treatment of the old and the ill without changing fundamental emotional attitudes and social relations. The topics must, therefore, be treated separately. In the next part of the discussion, nothing will be said about the social consequences and possible abuses of the practice of euthanasia, but only about acts of euthanasia considered in themselves.

What we want to know is whether acts of euthanasia, defined as we have defined them, are ever morally permissible. To be more accurate, we want to know whether it is ever sufficient justification of the choice of death for another that death can be counted a benefit rather than harm, and that this is why the choice is made.

It will be impossible to get a clear view of the area to which this topic belongs without first marking the distinct grounds on which objection may lie when one man opts for the death of another. There are two different virtues whose requirements are, in general, contrary to such actions. An unjustified act of killing, or allowing to die, is contrary to justice or to charity, or to both virtues, and the moral failings are distinct. Justice has to do with what men *owe* each other in the way of noninterference and positive service. When used in this wide sense, which has its history in the doctrine of the cardinal virtues, justice is not especially connected with, for instance, law courts but with the whole area of rights, and duties corresponding to rights. Thus murder is one form of injustice, dishonesty another, and wrongful failure to keep contracts a third; chicanery in a law court or defrauding someone of his inheritance are simply other cases of injustice. Justice as such is not directly linked to the good of another, and may require that something be rendered to him even where it will do him harm, as Hume pointed out when he remarked that a debt must be paid even to a profligate debauchee who "would rather receive harm than benefit from large possessions."[7] Charity, on the other hand, is the virtue which attaches us to the good of others. An act of charity is in question only where something is not demanded by justice, but a lack of charity and of justice can be shown where a man is denied something which he both needs and has a right to; both charity and justice demand that widows and orphans are not defrauded, and the man who cheats them is neither charitable nor just.

It is easy to see that the two grounds of objection to inducing death are distinct. A murder is an act of injustice. A culpable failure to come to the aid of someone whose life is threatened is normally contrary, not to justice, but to charity. But where one man is under contract, explicit or implicit, to come to the aid of another injustice too will be shown. Thus injustice may be involved either in an act or an omission, and the same is true of a lack of charity; charity may demand that someone be aided, but also that an unkind word not be spoken.

The distinction between charity and justice will turn out to be of the first importance when voluntary and nonvoluntary euthanasia are distinguished later on. This is because of the connection between justice and rights, and something should now be said about this. I believe it is true to say that wherever a man acts unjustly he has infringed a right, since justice has to do with whatever a man is owed, and whatever he is owed is his as a matter of right. Something should

7. David Hume, *Treatise*, Book III, Part II, Section 1.

Euthanasia

therefore be said about the different kinds of rights. The distinction commonly made is between having a right in the sense of having a liberty, and having a "claim-right" or "right of recipience."[8] The best way to understand such a distinction seems to be as follows. To say that a man has a right in the sense of a liberty is to say that no one can demand that he do not do the thing which he has a right to do. The fact that he has a right to do it consists in the fact that a certain kind of objection does not lie against his doing it. Thus a man has a right in this sense to walk down a public street or park his car in a public parking space. It does not follow that no one else may prevent him from doing so. If for some reason I want a certain man not to park in a certain place I may lawfully park there myself or get my friends to do so, thus preventing him from doing what he has a right (in the sense of a liberty) to do. It is different, however, with a claim-right. This is the kind of right which I have in addition to a liberty when, for example, I have a private parking space; now others have duties in the way of noninterference, as in this case, or of service, as in the case where my claim-right is to goods or services promised to me. Sometimes one of these rights gives other people the duty of securing to me that to which I have a right, but at other times their duty is merely to refrain from interference. If a fall of snow blocks my private parking space there is normally no obligation for anyone else to clear it away. Claim rights generate duties; sometimes these duties are duties of noninterference; sometimes they are duties of service. If your right gives me the duty not to interfere with you I have "no right" to do it; similarly, if your right gives me the duty to provide something for you I have "no right" to refuse to do it. What *I* lack is the right which is a liberty; I am not "at liberty" to interfere with you or to refuse the service.

Where in this picture does the right to life belong? No doubt people have the right to live in the sense of a liberty, but what is important is the cluster of claim-rights brought together under the title of the

8. See, for example D.D. Raphael, "Human Rights Old and New," in D.D. Raphael, ed., *Political Theory and the Rights of Man* (London, 1967), and Joel Feinberg, "The Nature and Value of Rights," *The Journal of Value Inquiry* 4, no. 4 (Winter 1970): 243–257. Reprinted in Samuel Gorovitz, ed., *Moral Problems in Medicine* (Englewood Cliffs, New Jersey, 1976).

right to life. The chief of these is, of course, the right to be free from interferences that threaten life. If other people aim their guns at us or try to pour poison into our drink we can, to put it mildly, demand that they desist. And then there are the services we can claim from doctors, health officers, bodyguards, and firemen; the rights that depend on contract or public arrangement. Perhaps there is no particular point in saying that the duties these people owe us belong to the right to life; we might as well say that all the services owed to anyone by tailors, dressmakers, and couturiers belong to a right called the right to be elegant. But contracts such as those understood in the patient-doctor relationship come in an important way when we are discussing the rights and wrongs of euthanasia, and are therefore mentioned here.

Do people have the right to what they need in order to survive, apart from the right conferred by special contracts into which other people have entered for the supplying of these necessities? Do people in the underdeveloped countries in which starvation is rife have the right to the food they so evidently lack? Joel Feinberg, discussing this question, suggests that they should be said to have "a claim," distinguishing this from a "valid claim," which gives a claim-right.

> The manifesto writers on the other side who seem to identify needs, or at least basic needs, with what they call "human rights," are more properly described, I think, as urging upon the world community the moral principle that *all* basic human needs ought to be recognized as *claims* (in the customary *prima facie* sense) worthy of sympathy and serious consideration right now, even though, in many cases, they cannot yet plausibly be treated as *valid* claims, that is, as grounds of any other people's duties. This way of talking avoids the anomaly of ascribing to all human beings now, even those in pre-industrial societies, such "economic and social rights" as "periodic holidays with pay."[9]

This seems reasonable, though we notice that there are some actual rights to service which are not based on anything like a contract, as for instance the right that children have to support from their parents and parents to support from their children in old age, though both

9. Feinberg, "Human Rights," *Moral Problems in Medicine*, p. 465.

sets of rights are to some extent dependent on existing social arrangements.

Let us now ask how the right to life affects the morality of acts of euthanasia. Are such acts sometimes or always ruled out by the right to life? This is certainly a possibility; for although an act of euthanasia is, by our definition, a matter of opting for death for the good of the one who is to die, there is, as we noted earlier, no direct connection between that to which a man has a right and that which is for his good. It is true that men have the right only to the kind of thing that is, in general, a good: we do not think that people have the right to garbage or polluted air. Nevertheless, a man may have the right to something which he himself would be better off without; where rights exist it is a man's will that counts not his or anyone else's estimate of benefit or harm. So the duties complementary to the right to life—the general duty of noninterference and the duty of service incurred by certain persons—are not affected by the quality of a man's life or by his prospects. Even if it is true that he would be, as we say, "better off dead," so long as he wants to live this does not justify us in killing him and may not justify us in deliberately allowing him to die. All of us have the duty of noninterference, and some of us may have the duty to sustain his life. Suppose, for example, that a retreating army has to leave behind wounded or exhausted soldiers in the wastes of an arid or snowbound land where the only prospect is death by starvation or at the hands of an enemy notoriously cruel. It has often been the practice to accord a merciful bullet to men in such desperate straits. But suppose that one of them demands that he should be left alive? It seems clear that his comrades have no right to kill him, though it is a quite different question as to whether they should give him a life-prolonging drug. The right to life can sometimes give a duty of positive service, but does not do so here. What it does give is the right to be left alone.

Interestingly enough we have arrived by way of a consideration of the right to life at the distinction normally labeled "active" versus "passive" euthanasia, and often thought to be irrelevant to the moral issue.[10] Once it is seen that the right to life is a distinct ground of

10. See, for example, James Rachels, "Active and Passive Euthanasia," *New England Journal of Medicine* 292, no. 2 (9 Jan. 1975): 78–80.

objection to certain acts of euthanasia, and that this right creates a duty of noninterference more widespread than the duties of care there can be no doubt about the relevance of the distinction between passive and active euthanasia. Where everyone may have the duty to leave someone alone, it may be that no one has the duty to maintain his life, or that only some people do.

Where then do the boundaries of the "active" and "passive" lie? In some ways the words are themselves misleading, because they suggest the difference between act and omission which is not quite what we want. Certainly the act of shooting someone is the kind of thing we were talking about under the heading of "interference," and omitting to give him a drug a case of refusing care. But the act of turning off a respirator should surely be thought of as no different from the decision not to start it; if doctors had decided that a patient should be allowed to die, either course of action might follow, and both should be counted as passive rather than active euthanasia if euthanasia were in question. The point seems to be that interference in a course of treatment is not the same as other interference in a man's life, and particularly if the same body of people are responsible for the treatment and for its discontinuance. In such a case we could speak of the disconnecting of the apparatus as killing the man, or of the hospital as allowing him to die. By and large, it is the act of killing that is ruled out under the heading of noninterference, but not in every case.

Doctors commonly recognize this distinction, and the grounds on which some philosophers have denied it seem untenable. James Rachels, for instance, believes that if the difference between active and passive is relevant anywhere, it should be relevant everywhere, and he has pointed to an example in which it seems to make no difference which is done. If someone saw a child drowning in a bath it would seem just as bad to let it drown as to push its head under water.[11] If "it makes no difference" means that one act would be as iniquitous as the other this is true. It is not that killing is *worse* than allowing to die, but that the two are contrary to distinct virtues, which gives the possibility that in some circumstances one is impermissible and the other permissible. In the circumstances invented by Rachels, both are

11. Ibid.

wicked: it is contrary to justice to push the child's head under the water—something one has no right to do. To leave it to drown is not contrary to justice, but it is a particularly glaring example of lack of charity. Here it makes no practical difference because the requirements of justice and charity coincide; but in the case of the retreating army they did not: charity would have required that the wounded soldier be killed had not justice required that he be left alive.[12] In such a case it makes all the difference whether a man opts for the death of another in a positive action, or whether he allows him to die. An analogy with the right to property will make the point clear. If a man owns something he has the right to it even when its possession does him harm, and we have no right to take it from him. But if one day it should blow away, maybe nothing requires us to get it back for him; we could not deprive him of it, but we may allow it to go. This is not to deny that it will often be an unfriendly act or one based on an arrogant judgment when we refuse to do what he wants. Nevertheless, we would be within our rights, and it might be that no moral objection of any kind would lie against our refusal.

It is important to emphasize that a man's rights may stand between us and the action we would dearly like to take for his sake. They may, of course, also prevent action which we would like to take for the sake of others, as when it might be tempting to kill one man to save several. But it is interesting that the limits of allowable interference, however uncertain, seem stricter in the first case than the second. Perhaps there are no cases in which it would be all right to kill a man against his will *for his own sake* unless they could equally well be described as cases of allowing him to die, as in the example of turning off the respirator. However, there are circumstances, even if these are very rare, in which one man's life would justifiably be sacrificed to save others, and "killing" would be the only description of what was being done. For instance, a vehicle which had gone out of control might be steered from a path on which it would kill more than one man to a path on which it would kill one.[13] But it would not be permissible to

12. It is not, however, that justice and charity conflict. A man does not lack charity because he refrains from an act of injustice which would have been for someone's good.

13. For a discussion of such questions, see my article "The Problem of Abortion and the Doctrine of Double Effect," *Oxford Review*, no. 5 (1967); reprinted in Rachels, *Moral Problems*, and Gorovitz, *Moral Problems in Medicine*.

steer a vehicle towards someone in order to kill him, against his will, for his own good. An analogy with property rights illustrates the point. One may not destroy a man's property against his will on the grounds that he would be better off without it; there are however circumstances in which it could be destroyed for the sake of others. If his house is liable to fall and kill him that is his affair; it might, however, without injustice be destroyed to stop the spread of a fire.

We see then that the distinction between active and passive, important as it is elsewhere, has a special importance in the area of euthanasia. It should also be clear why James Rachels' other argument, that it is often "more humane" to kill than to allow to die, does not show that the distinction between active and passive euthanasia is morally irrelevant. It might be "more humane" in this sense to deprive a man of the property that brings evils on him, or to refuse to pay what is owed to Hume's profligate debauchee; but if we say this we must admit that an act which is "more humane" than its alternative may be morally objectionable because it infringes rights.

So far we have said very little about the right to service as opposed to the right to noninterference, though it was agreed that both might be brought under the heading of "the right to life." What about the duty to preserve life that may belong to special classes of persons such as bodyguards, firemen, or doctors? Unlike the general public they are not within their rights if they merely refrain from interfering and do not try to sustain life. The subject's claim-rights are two-fold as far as they are concerned and passive as well as active euthanasia may be ruled out here if it is against his will. This is not to say that he has the right to any and every service needed to save or prolong his life; the rights of other people set limits to what may be demanded, both because they have the right not to be interfered with and because they may have a competing right to services. Furthermore one must enquire just what the contract or implicit agreement amounts to in each case. Firemen and bodyguards presumably have a duty which is simply to preserve life, within the limits of justice to others and of reasonableness to themselves. With doctors it may however be different, since their duty relates not only to preserving life but also to the relief of suffering. It is not clear what a doctor's duties are to his patient if life can be prolonged only at the cost of suffering or suffering relieved only by measures that shorten life. George Fletcher has argued that what the doctor is under contract to do depends on what is generally done, because this is what a patient will reasonably expect.[11] This seems right. If procedures are part of normal medical practice then it seems that the patient can demand them however much it may be against his interest to do do. Once again it is not a matter of what is "most humane."

That the patient's right to life may set limits to permissible acts of euthanasia seems undeniable. If he does not want to die no one has the right to practice active euthanasia on him, and passive euthanasia may also be ruled out where he has a right to the services of doctors or others.

Perhaps few will deny what has so far been said about the impermissibility of acts of euthanasia simply because we have so far spoken about the case of one who positively wants to live, and about his rights, whereas those who advocate euthanasia are usually thinking either about those who wish to die or about those whose wishes cannot be ascertained either because they cannot properly be said to have wishes or because, for one reason or another, we are unable to form a reliable estimate of what they are. The question that must now be asked is whether the latter type of case, where euthanasia though not involuntary would again be nonvoluntary, is different from the one discussed so far. Would we have the right to kill someone for his own good so long as we had no idea that he positively wished to live? And what about the life-prolonging duties of doctors in the same circumstances? This is a very difficult problem. On the one hand, it seems ridiculous to suppose that a man's right to life is something which generates duties only where he has signaled that he wants to live; as a borrower does indeed have a duty to return something lent on indefinite loan only if the lender indicates that he wants it back. On the other hand, it might be argued that there is something illogical about the idea that a right has been infringed if someone incapable of saying whether he wants it or not is deprived of something that is doing him harm rather than good. Yet on the analogy of property we would say that a right has been infringed. Only if someone had earlier

14. George Fletcher, "Legal Aspects of the Decision not to Prolong Life," *Journal of the American Medical Association* 203, no. 1 (1 Jan. 1968): 119–122. Reprinted in Gorovitz.

told us that in such circumstances he would not want to keep the
thing could we think that his right had been waived. Perhaps if we
could make confident judgments about what anyone in such circumstances would wish, or what he would have wished beforehand had he
considered the matter, we could agree to consider the right to life as
"dormant," needing to be asserted if the normal duties were to remain.
But as things are we cannot make any such assumption; we simply
do not know what most people would want, or would have wanted,
us to do unless they tell us. This is certainly the case so far as active
measures to end life are concerned. Possibly it is different, or will
become different, in the matter of being kept alive, so general is the
feeling against using sophisticated procedures on moribund patients,
and so much is this dreaded by people who are old or terminally ill.
Once again the distinction between active and passive euthanasia has
come on the scene, but this time because most people's attitudes to the
two are so different. It is just possible that we might presume, in the
absence of specific evidence, that someone would not wish, beyond a
certain point, to be kept alive; it is certainly not possible to assume
that he would wish to be killed.

In the last paragraph we have begun to broach the topic of voluntary euthanasia, and this we must now discuss. What is to be said
about the case in which there is no doubt about someone's wish to
die: either he has told us beforehand that he would wish it in circumstances such as he is now in, and has shown no sign of a change of
mind, or else he tells us now, being in possession of his faculties and
of a steady mind. We should surely say that the objections previously
urged against acts of euthanasia, which it must be remembered were
all on the ground of rights, had disappeared. It does not seem that one
would infringe someone's right to life in killing him with his permission and in fact at his request. Why should someone not be able to
waive his right to life, or rather, as would be more likely to happen,
to cancel some of the duties of noninterference that this right entails?
(He is more likely to say that he should be killed by this man at this
time in this manner, than to say that anyone may kill him at any time
and in any way.) Similarly someone may give permission for the
destruction of his property, and request it. The important thing is
that he gives a critical permission, and it seems that this is enough

to cancel the duty normally associated with the right. If someone gives you permission to destroy his property it can no longer be said that you have no right to do so, and I do not see why it should not be the case with taking a man's life. An objection might be made on the ground that only God has the right to take life, but in this paper religious as opposed to moral arguments are being left aside. Religion apart, there seems to be no case to be made out for an infringement of rights if a man who wishes to die is allowed to die or even killed. But of course it does not follow that there is no moral objection to it. Even with property, which is after all a relatively small matter, one might be wrong to destroy what one had the right to destroy. For, apart from its value to other people, it might be valuable to the man who wanted it destroyed, and charity might require us to hold our hand where justice did not.

Let us review the conclusion of this part of the argument, which has been about euthanasia and the right to life. It has been argued that from this side come stringent restrictions on the acts of euthanasia that could be morally permissible. Active nonvoluntary euthanasia is ruled out by that part of the right to life which creates the duty of noninterference though passive nonvoluntary euthanasia is not ruled out, except where the right to life-preserving action has been created by some special condition such as a contract between a man and his doctor, and it is not always certain just what such a contract involves. Voluntary euthanasia is another matter: as the preceding paragraph suggested, no right is infringed if a man is allowed to die or even killed at his own request.

Turning now to the other objection that normally holds against inducing the death of another, that it is against charity, or benevolence, we must tell a very different story. Charity is the virtue that gives attachment to the good of others, and because life is normally a good, charity normally demands that it should be saved or prolonged. But as we so defined an act of euthanasia that it seeks a man's death for his own sake—for his good—charity will normally speak in favor of it. This is not, of course, to say that charity can require an act of euthanasia which justice forbids, but if an act of euthanasia is not contrary to justice—that is, it does not infringe rights—charity will rather be in its favor than against.

Once more the distinction between nonvoluntary and voluntary euthanasia must be considered. Could it ever be compatible with charity to seek a man's death although he wanted to live, or at least had not let us know that he wanted to die? It has been argued that in such circumstances active euthanasia would infringe his right to life, but passive euthanasia would not do so, unless he had some special right to life-preserving service from the one who allowed him to die. What would charity dictate? Obviously when a man wants to live there is a presumption that he will be benefited if his life is prolonged, and if it is so the question of euthanasia does not arise. But it is, on the other hand, possible that he wants to live where it would be better for him to die: perhaps he does not realize the desperate situation he is in, or perhaps he is afraid of dying. So, in spite of a very proper resistance to refusing to go along with a man's own wishes in the matter of life and death, someone might justifiably refuse to prolong the life even of someone who asked him to prolong it, as in the case of refusing to give the wounded soldier a drug that would keep him alive to meet a terrible end. And it is even more obvious that charity does not always dictate that life should be prolonged where a man's own wishes, hypothetical or actual, are not known.

So much for the relation of charity to nonvoluntary passive euthanasia, which was not, like nonvoluntary active euthanasia, ruled out by the right to life. Let us now ask what charity has to say about voluntary euthanasia both active and passive. It was suggested in the discussion of justice that if of sound mind and steady desire a man might give others the *right* to allow him to die or even to kill him, where otherwise this would be ruled out. But it was pointed out that this would not settle the question of whether the act was morally permissible, and it is this that we must now consider. Could not charity speak against what justice allowed? Indeed it might do so. For while the fact that a man wants to die suggests that his life is wretched, and while his rejection of life may itself tend to take the good out of the things he might have enjoyed, nevertheless his wish to die might here be opposed for his own sake just as it might be if suicide were in question. Perhaps there is hope that his mental condition will improve. Perhaps he is mistaken in thinking his disease incurable. Perhaps he wants to die for the sake of someone else on whom he feels he is a burden, and we are not ready to accept this sacrifice whether for ourselves or others. In such cases, and there will surely be many of them, it could not be for his own sake that we kill him or allow him to die, and therefore euthanasia as defined in this paper would not be in question. But this is not to deny that there could be acts of voluntary euthanasia both passive and active against which neither justice nor charity would speak.

We have now considered the morality of euthanasia both voluntary and nonvoluntary, and active and passive. The conclusion has been that nonvoluntary active euthanasia (roughly, killing a man against his will or without his consent) is never justified; that is to say, that a man's being killed for his own good never justifies the act unless he himself has consented to it. A man's rights are infringed by such an action, and it is therefore contrary to justice. However, all the other combinations, nonvoluntary passive euthanasia, voluntary active euthanasia, and voluntary passive euthanasia are sometimes compatible with both justice and charity. But the strong condition carried in the definition of euthanasia adopted in this paper must not be forgotten; an act of euthanasia as here understood is one whose purpose is to benefit the one who dies.

In the light of this discussion let us look at our present practices. Are they good or are they bad? And what changes might be made, thinking now not only of the morality of particular acts of euthanasia but also of the indirect effects of instituting different practices, of the abuses to which they might be subject and of the changes that might come about if euthanasia became a recognized part of the social scene.

The first thing to notice is that it is wrong to ask whether we should introduce the practice of euthanasia as if it were not something we already had. In fact we do have it. For instance it is common, where the medical prognosis is very bad, for doctors to recommend against measures to prolong life, and particularly where a process of degeneration producing one medical emergency after another has already set in. If these doctors are not certainly within their legal rights this is something that is apt to come as a surprise to them as to the general public. It is also obvious that euthanasia is often practiced where old people are concerned. If someone very old and soon to die is attacked by a disease that makes his life wretched, doctors do not always come in with life-prolonging drugs. Perhaps poor patients are more fortunate in this respect than rich patients, being more often left to die in peace; but it is in any case a well recognized piece of medical practice, which is a form of euthanasia.

No doubt the case of infants with mental or physical defects will be suggested as another example of the practice of euthanasia as we already have it, since such infants are sometimes deliberately allowed to die. That they are deliberately allowed to die is certain; children with severe spina bifida malformations are not always operated on even where it is thought that without the operation they will die; and even in the case of children with Down's Syndrome who have intestinal obstructions the relatively simple operation that would make it possible to feed them is sometimes not performed.[15] Whether this is euthanasia in our sense or only as the Nazis understood it is another matter. We must ask the crucial question, "Is it for the sake of the child himself that the doctors and parents choose his death?" In some cases the answer may really be yes, and what is more important it may really be true that the kind of life which is a good is not possible or likely for this child, and that there is little but suffering and frustration in store for him.[16] But this must presuppose that the medical prognosis is wretchedly bad, as it may be for some spina bifida children. With children who are born with Down's Syndrome it is, however, quite different. Most of these are able to live on for quite a time in a reasonably contented way, remaining like children all their lives but capable of affectionate relationships and able to play games and perform simple tasks. The fact is, of course, that the doctors who recommend against life-saving procedures for handicapped infants are usually thinking not of them but rather of their parents and of other children in the family or of the "burden on society" if the chil-

15. I have been told this by a pediatrician in a well-known medical center in the United States. It is confirmed by Anthony M. Shaw and Iris A. Shaw, "Dilemma of Informed Consent in Children," *The New England Journal of Medicine* 289, no. 17 (25 Oct. 1973): 885–890. Reprinted in Gorovitz.

16. It must be remembered, however, that many of the social miseries of spina bifida children could be avoided. Professor R.B. Zachary is surely right to insist on this. See, for example, "Ethical and Social Aspects of Spina Bifida," *The Lancet*, 3 Aug. 1968, pp. 274–276. Reprinted in Gorovitz.

dren survive. So it is not for their sake but to avoid trouble to others that they are allowed to die. When brought out into the open this seems unacceptable: at least we do not easily accept the principle that adults who need special care should be counted too burdensome to be kept alive. It must in any case be insisted that if children with Down's Syndrome are deliberately allowed to die this is not a matter of euthanasia except in Hitler's sense. And for our children, since we scruple to gas them, not even the manner of their death is "quiet and easy"; when not treated for an intestinal obstruction a baby simply starves to death. Perhaps some will take this as an argument for allowing active euthanasia, in which case they will be in the company of an S.S. man stationed in the Warthgenau who sent Eichmann a memorandum telling him that "Jews in the coming winter could no longer be fed" and submitting for his consideration a proposal as to whether "it would not be the most humane solution to kill those Jews who were incapable of work through some quicker means."[17] If we say we are *unable* to look after children with handicaps we are no more telling the truth than was the S.S. man who said that the Jews could not be fed.

Nevertheless if it is ever right to allow deformed children to die because life will be a misery to them, or not to take measures to prolong for a little the life of a newborn baby whose life cannot extend beyond a few months of intense medical intervention, there is a genuine problem about active as opposed to passive euthanasia. There are well-known cases in which the medical staff has looked on wretchedly while an infant died slowly from starvation and dehydration because they did not feel able to give a lethal injection. According to the principles discussed in the earlier part of this paper they would indeed have had no right to give it, since an infant cannot ask that it should be done. The only possible solution—supposing that voluntary active euthanasia were to be legalized—would be to appoint guardians to act on the infant's behalf. In a different climate of opinion this might not be dangerous, but at present, when people so readily assume that the life of a handicapped baby is of no value, one would be loath to support it.

Finally, on the subject of handicapped children, another word

17. Quoted by Hannah Arendt, *Eichmann in Jerusalem* (London, 1963), p. 90.

should be said about those with severe mental defects. For them too it might sometimes be right to say that one would wish for death for their sake. But not even severe mental handicap automatically brings a child within the scope even of a possible act of euthanasia. If the level of consciousness is low enough it could not be said that life is a good to them, any more than in the case of those suffering from extreme senility. Nevertheless if they do not suffer it will not be an act of euthanasia by which someone opts for their death. Perhaps charity does not demand that strenuous measures are taken to keep people in this state alive, but euthanasia does not come into the matter, any more than it does when someone is, like Karen Ann Quinlan, in a state of permanent coma. Much could be said about this last case. It might even be suggested that in the case of unconsciousness this "life" is not the life to which "the right to life" refers. But that is not our topic here.

What we must consider, even if only briefly, is the possibility that euthanasia, genuine euthanasia, and not contrary to the requirements of justice or charity, should be legalized over a wider area. Here we are up against the really serious problem of abuse. Many people want, and want very badly, to be rid of their elderly relatives and even of their ailing husbands or wives. Would any safeguards ever be able to stop them describing as euthanasia what was really for their own benefit? And would it be possible to prevent the occurrence of acts which were genuinely acts of euthanasia but morally impermissible because infringing the rights of a patient who wished to live?

Perhaps the furthest we should go is to encourage patients to make their own contracts with a doctor by making it known whether they wish him to prolong their life in case of painful terminal illness or of incapacity. A document such as the Living Will seems eminently sensible, and should surely be allowed to give a doctor following the previously expressed wishes of the patient immunity from legal proceedings by relatives.[18] Legalizing active euthanasia is, however, another matter. Apart from the special repugnance doctors feel

18. Details of this document are to be found in J.A. Behnke and Sissela Bok, eds., *The Dilemmas of Euthanasia* (New York, 1975), and in A.B. Downing, ed., *Euthanasia and the Right to Life: The Case for Voluntary Euthanasia* (London, 1969).

towards the idea of a lethal injection, it may be of the very greatest importance to keep a psychological barrier up against killing. Moreover it is active euthanasia which is the most liable to abuse. Hitler would not have been able to kill 275,000 people in his "euthanasia" program if he had had to wait for them to need life-saving treatment. But there are other objections to active euthanasia, even voluntary active euthanasia. In the first place it would be hard to devise procedures that would protect people from being persuaded into giving their consent. And secondly the possibility of active voluntary euthanasia might change the social scene in ways that would be very bad. As things are, people do, by and large, expect to be looked after if they are old or ill. This is one of the good things that we have, but we might lose it, and be much worse off without it. It might come to be expected that someone likely to need a lot of looking after should call for the doctor and demand his own death. Something comparable could be good in an extremely poverty-stricken community where the children genuinely suffered from lack of food; but in rich societies such as ours it would surely be a spiritual disaster. Such possibilities should make us very wary of supporting large measures of euthanasia, even where moral principle applied to the individual act does not rule it out.

THE CONTRIBUTORS

KENNETH J. ARROW is Joan Kenney Professor of Economics and Professor of Operations Research at Stanford University. His most recent book is *Studies in Resource Allocation Processes* (with Leonid Hurwicz). His current area of research is the role of information, uncertainty, and organization in economic behavior.

LAWRENCE C. BECKER, Professor of Philosophy at Hollins College, Virginia, is the author of *On Justifying Moral Judgments* (London: Routledge & Kegan Paul, 1973), *Property Rights: Philosophic Foundations* (London: Routledge & Kegan Paul, 1977), and articles in moral and legal philosophy.

CHRISTOPHER BOORSE, Associate Professor of Philosophy at the University of Delaware, works mainly in philosophy of language and philosophy of science. His article in this Reader is one of three he has written on the concept of health.

ALLEN BUCHANAN is Professor of Philosophy at the University of Arizona. He has published articles on the subjects of ethics, political philosophy, and epistemology. His book *Marx and Justice* (Rowman and Littlefield) will appear in the Spring of 1982.

CHARLES M. CULVER is Professor
of Psychiatry at Dartmouth Medical School. He obtained an M.D.
and a Ph.D. in Clinical Psychology
from Duke University. He is the
coauthor, with Bernard Gert, of
Philosophy in Medicine, which
will be published by Oxford
University Press in 1982.

NORMAN DANIELS is Professor of
Philosophy at Tufts University.
He is the author of *Thomas Reid's
'Inquiry'* (New York: Burt Frank-
lin, 1974), editor of *Reading
Rawls* (New York: Basic Books,
1975), and is currently working
on *Justice and Health Care Delivery*, to be published by Cambridge University Press.

JOEL FEINBERG is Professor of
Philosophy at The University of
Arizona. He is the author of *Doing
and Deserving* (Princeton Uni-
versity Press, 1970), *Social Phi-
losophy* (Englewood Cliffs, N.J.:
Prentice-Hall, 1973), and *Rights,
Justice, and the Bounds of Liberty*
(Princeton University Press,
1980).

MICHAEL B. GREEN, who holds
doctorates in both philosophy and
clinical psychology, is in private
practice in Los Angeles. He has
published articles in philosophy
of mind, psychology, ethics, and
medical ethics.

PHILIPPA FOOT is Professor of
Philosophy at the University of
California, Los Angeles and Senior
Research Fellow at Somerville
College, Oxford. She is the author
of *Virtues and Vices and other
Essays in Moral Philosophy* (University of California Press, 1978).

BERNARD GERT is Stone Professor
of Intellectual and Moral Philosophy at Dartmouth College and
Adjunct Professor of Psychiatry
at Dartmouth Medical School. He
is the author of *The Moral Rules*,
3d ed. (New York: Harper &
Row, 1975), editor of *Man and
Citizen* by Thomas Hobbes (New
York: Anchor Books, 1972) and
coauthor (with Charles M. Culver)
of *Philosophy in Medicine* (New
York: Oxford University Press,
1982). He s currently a recipient
of a NEH-NSF Sustained Development Award.

LOREN E. LOMASKY is Associate
Professor and Chairman of the
Department of Philosophy, University of Minnesota, Duluth. He
has published articles in ethics
and the philosophy of religion,
and is presently writing a book on
the foundations of human rights
theory.

JAMES L. MUYSKENS is Associate
Professor of Philosophy at Hunter
College, The City University of
New York. He is author of *The
Sufficiency of Hope* (Philadelphia:
Temple University Press, 1979)
and *Moral Problems in Nursing*,
which will be published by Rowman and Littlefield in 1982.

PETER SINGER is Professor of Philosophy at Monash University, Melbourne, Australia. His books include *Animal Liberation* (New York: A New York Review Book, 1975); *Practical Ethics* (Cambridge: Cambridge University Press, 1979); and *The Expanding Circle: Ethics and Sociobiology* (New York: Farrar, Straus & Giroux, 1981). He is now working with the Monash University Center for Human Bioethics on the ethics of life and death choices for defective newborns.

STEPHEN P. STICH is Professor of Philosophy at the University of Maryland. He is the editor of *Innate Ideas* (University of California Press, 1975) and coeditor with David A. Jackson of *The Recombinant DNA Debate* (Englewood Cliffs, N.J.: Prentice-Hall, 1979). His new book, *The Case Against Belief*, will be published by MIT Press.

DONALD VANDEVEER is Professor of Philosophy at North Carolina State University. He has coedited an anthology, *And Justice for All*, and is writing a book tentatively entitled *Paternalism: Constraining Others for Their Own Good*.

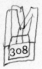

DANIEL WIKLER is Associate
Professor in the Program in Medical Ethics, Center for Health
Sciences, and in the Department
of Philosophy, both of the University of Wisconsin, Madison.
He is the author of "Paternalism
and the Mildly Retarded," which
appeared in *Philosophy & Public
Affairs*, and of other articles in
medical ethics. He was consultant
on philosophical issues in the
definition of death to both the
Wisconsin state legislature and
the President's Commission for
the Study of Ethical Problems
in Medicine, 1980-81, and is
currently working on a book
concerning the attempts by
government to resolve issues in
medical ethics.